NATIONAL
ACADEMIES

Sciences
Engineering
Medicine

TIONAL
ADEMIES
SS
hington, DC

Adult Attention-Deficit/ Hyperactivity Disorder

Diagnosis, Treatment, and Implications for Drug Development

Kelsey R. Babik, Noah Ontjes,
Carol Berkower,
Sheena M. Posey Norris, and
Carolyn Shore, *Rapporteurs*

Forum on Drug Discovery,
Development, and Translation

Forum on Neuroscience and Nervous
System Disorders

Board on Health Sciences Policy

Health and Medicine Division

Proceedings of a Workshop

NATIONAL ACADEMIES PRESS 500 Fifth Street, NW Washington, DC 20001

This activity was supported by contracts between the National Academy of Sciences and Acadia Pharmaceuticals; Alzheimer's Association; American Brain Coalition; American Neurological Association; Amgen Inc.; Association of American Medical Colleges; AstraZeneca; Biogen; Boehringer Ingelheim (Contract No. 755326); BrightFocus Foundation; Burroughs Wellcome Fund (Contract No. 1023129); California Institute for Regenerative Medicine; Cerevel Therapeutics; Cohen Veterans Bioscience; Department of Veteran Affairs (Contract No. 36C24E20C009); Eisai; Eli Lilly and Company; FasterCures, Milken Institute; Foundation for the National Institutes of Health; Friends of Cancer Research; Gatsby Charitable Foundation; Harmony Biosciences; Janssen Research & Development, LLC; Johnson & Johnson; Karuna Therapeutics; Lundbeck Research USA, Inc.; Medable Inc.; Merck & Co., Inc. (Contract No. MRLCPO-23-166623); Michael J. Fox Foundation for Parkinson's Research; National Institutes of Health (Contract No. HHSN263201800029I; Task Order Nos. HHSN26300007 and 75N98024F00001): BRAIN Initiative, National Cancer Institute, National Center for Advancing Translational Sciences, National Center for Complementary and Integrative Health, National Eye Institute, National Institute of Allergy and Infectious Diseases, National Institute of Environmental Health Sciences, National Institute of Mental Health, National Institute of Neurological Disorders and Stroke, National Institute on Aging, National Institute on Alcohol Abuse and Alcoholism, and National Institute on Drug Abuse, Office of the Director; National Multiple Sclerosis Society; National Science Foundation; New England Journal of Medicine; One Mind; Paul G. Allen Frontiers Group; Sanofi (Contract No. 77646387); Simons Foundation (Contract No. 995152); Takeda (Contract No. A62909); The George & Anne Ryan Institute for Neuroscience at the University of Rhode Island; U.S. Food and Drug Administration (Contract No. 1R13FD007302-01, Contract No. 1R13FD005362-01, and Contract No. 1R13FD008016); Wellcome Trust. Any opinions, findings, conclusions, or recommendations expressed in this publication do not necessarily reflect the views of any organization or agency that provided support for the project.

International Standard Book Number-13: 978-0-309-71916-2
International Standard Book Number-10: 0-309-71916-X
Digital Object Identifier: https://doi.org/10.17226/27770

This publication is available from the National Academies Press, 500 Fifth Street, NW, Keck 360, Washington, DC 20001; (800) 624-6242 or (202) 334-3313; http://www.nap.edu.

Suggested citation: National Academies of Sciences, Engineering, and Medicine. 2024. *Adult attention-deficit/hyperactivity disorder: Diagnosis, treatment, and implications for drug development: Proceedings of a workshop.* Washington, DC: The National Academies Press. https://doi.org/10.17226/27770.

The **National Academy of Sciences** was established in 1863 by an Act of Congress, signed by President Lincoln, as a private, nongovernmental institution to advise the nation on issues related to science and technology. Members are elected by their peers for outstanding contributions to research. Dr. Marcia McNutt is president.

The **National Academy of Engineering** was established in 1964 under the charter of the National Academy of Sciences to bring the practices of engineering to advising the nation. Members are elected by their peers for extraordinary contributions to engineering. Dr. John L. Anderson is president.

The **National Academy of Medicine** (formerly the Institute of Medicine) was established in 1970 under the charter of the National Academy of Sciences to advise the nation on medical and health issues. Members are elected by their peers for distinguished contributions to medicine and health. Dr. Victor J. Dzau is president.

The three Academies work together as the **National Academies of Sciences, Engineering, and Medicine** to provide independent, objective analysis and advice to the nation and conduct other activities to solve complex problems and inform public policy decisions. The National Academies also encourage education and research, recognize outstanding contributions to knowledge, and increase public understanding in matters of science, engineering, and medicine.

Learn more about the National Academies of Sciences, Engineering, and Medicine at **www.nationalacademies.org**.

PLANNING COMMITTEE FOR A WORKSHOP ON ADULT ATTENTION-DEFICIT/HYPERACTIVITY DISORDER (ADHD): DIAGNOSIS, TREATMENT, AND IMPLICATIONS FOR DRUG DEVELOPMENT[1]

CARLOS BLANCO (*Co-Chair*), Director, Division of Epidemiology, Services, and Prevention Research, National Institute on Drug Abuse
CRAIG B. H. SURMAN (*Co-Chair*), Director, Clinical and Research Program in Adult ADHD, Massachusetts General Hospital; Associate Professor of Psychiatry, Harvard Medical School
AMY F. T. ARNSTEN, Albert E. Kent Professor of Neuroscience and Professor of Psychology, Yale University School of Medicine
ANDREA M. CHRONIS-TUSCANO, Joel and Kim Feller Professor of Psychology and Director of the SUCCEEDS: Students Understanding College Choices, Encouraging and Executing Decisions for Success program, University of Maryland, College Park
TALEED EL-SABAWI, Assistant Professor of Law, Florida International University; Visiting Assistant Professor of Law, St. Louis University School of Law; Research Scholar, O'Neill Institute for National and Global Health Law, Georgetown Law Center
EVELYN POLK GREEN, Immediate Past President, Attention Deficit Disorder Association; Past President, Children and Adults with ADHD
STEVE S. LEE, Professor of Psychology, Director of Clinical Psychology Training, University of California, Los Angeles
JAMES (JIMMY) LEONARD, Director Clinical Services, Maryland Poison Center; Associate Professor, University of Maryland School of Pharmacy
TAMARA ROSIER, Founder, ADHD Center of West Michigan; President, ADHD Coaches Organization
MATTHEW RUDORFER, Chief, Psychopharmacology, Somatic, and Integrated Treatment Research Program, National Institute of Mental Health
ALMUT G. WINTERSTEIN, Distinguished Professor of Pharmaceutical Outcomes and Policy, Director of the Center for Drug Evaluation and Safety, University of Florida
STEVIN H. ZORN, President and Chief Executive Officer, MindImmune Therapeutics, Inc.

---

[1] The National Academies of Sciences, Engineering, and Medicine's planning committees are solely responsible for organizing the workshop, identifying topics, and choosing speakers. The responsibility for the published Proceedings of a Workshop rests with the workshop rapporteurs and the institution.

FORUM ON DRUG DISCOVERY, DEVELOPMENT, AND TRANSLATION[1]

GREGORY SIMON (*Co-Chair*), Kaiser Permanente Washington Health Research Institute; University of Washington
ANN TAYLOR (*Co-Chair*), Retired
BARBARA E. BIERER, Harvard Medical School; Brigham and Women's Hospital
LINDA BRADY, National Institute of Mental Health, NIH
JOHN BUSE, University of North Carolina, Chapel Hill School of Medicine
LUTHER T. CLARK, Merck & Co., Inc.
BARRY S. COLLER, The Rockefeller University
TAMMY R. L. COLLINS, Burroughs Wellcome Fund
THOMAS CURRAN, Children's Mercy, Kansas City
RICHARD DAVEY, National Institute of Allergy and Infectious Diseases, NIH
KATHERINE DAWSON, Biogen
JAMES H. DOROSHOW, National Cancer Institute, NIH
JEFFREY M. DRAZEN, *New England Journal of Medicine*
STEVEN K. GALSON, Retired
CARLOS O. GARNER, Eli Lilly and Company
SALLY L. HODDER, West Virginia University
TESHEIA JOHNSON, Yale School of Medicine
LYRIC JORGENSON, Office of the Director, NIH
ESTHER KROFAH, FasterCures, Milken Institute
LISA M. LaVANGE, University of North Carolina
ARAN MAREE, Johnson & Johnson
CRISTIAN MASSACESI, AstraZeneca
ROSS McKINNEY JR., Association of American Medical Colleges
JOSEPH P. MENETSKI, Foundation for the National Institutes of Health
ANAEZE C. OFFODILE II, Memorial Sloan Kettering Center
SALLY OKUN, Clinical Trials Transformation Initiative
ARTI RAI, Duke University School of Law
KLAUS ROMERO, Critical Path Institute
JONI RUTTER, National Center for Advancing Translational Sciences, NIH
SUSAN SCHAEFFER, The Patients' Academy for Research Advocacy
ANANTHA SHEKHAR, University of Pittsburgh School of Medicine

---

[1] The National Academies of Sciences, Engineering, and Medicine's forums and roundtables do not issue, review, or approve individual documents. The responsibility for the published Proceedings of a Workshop rests with the workshop rapporteurs and the institution.

ELLEN V. SIGAL, Friends of Cancer Research
MARK TAISEY, Amgen Inc.
AMIR TAMIZ, National Institute of Neurological Disorders and Stroke, NIH
PAMELA TENAERTS, Medable Inc.
JONATHAN WATANABE, University of California, Irvine School of Pharmacy and Pharmaceutical Sciences
ALASTAIR WOOD, Vanderbilt University
CRIS WOOLSTON, Sanofi
JOSEPH C. WU, Stanford University School of Medicine

Forum Staff

CAROLYN SHORE, Director, Forum on Drug Discovery, Development, and Translation
KYLE CAVAGNINI, Associate Program Officer
BRITTANY HSIAO, Associate Program Officer (*until March 2024*)
NOAH ONTJES, Associate Program Officer (*starting February 2024*)
MELVIN JOPPY, Senior Program Assistant
CLARE STROUD, Senior Director, Board on Health Sciences Policy

FORUM ON NEUROSCIENCE AND NERVOUS SYSTEM DISORDERS[1]

FRANCES JENSEN (*Co-Chair*), University of Pennsylvania
JOHN KRYSTAL (*Co-Chair*), Yale University
RITA BALICE-GORDON, Muna Therapeutics
DEANNA BARCH, Washington University in St. Louis
DIANE BOVENKAMP, BrightFocus Foundation (*as of August 2023*)
KATJA BROSE, Chan Zuckerberg Initiative
TERESA BURACCHIO, Food and Drug Administration
SARAH CADDICK, The Gatsby Charitable Foundation
ROSA CANET-AVILÉS, California Institute for Regenerative Medicine (CIRM)
MARIA CARRILLO, Alzheimer's Association
MICHAEL CHIANG, National Eye Institute
TIM COETZEE, National Multiple Sclerosis Society
BEVERLY DAVIDSON, University of Pennsylvania
NITA FARAHANY, Duke University
EVA FELDMAN, University of Michigan
BRIAN FISKE, The Michael J. Fox Foundation for Parkinson's Research
JOSHUA GORDON, National Institute of Mental Health
MORTEN GRUNNET, Lundbeck
MAGALI HAAS, Cohen Veterans Bioscience
RICHARD HODES, National Institute on Aging
STUART HOFFMAN, Department of Veterans Affairs
YASMIN HURD, Icahn School of Medicine at Mount Sinai
STEVEN HYMAN, The Broad Institute of MIT and Harvard
MICHAEL IRIZARRY, Eisai Inc.
GEORGE KOOB, National Institute on Alcohol Abuse and Alcoholism
WALTER KOROSHETZ, National Institute of Neurological Disorders and Stroke
ROBERT MALENKA, Stanford University
HUSSEINI MANJI, Oxford University; Duke University; UK Government Mental Health Mission
HUGH MARSTON, Boehringer Ingelheim
BILL MARTIN, Janssen Research & Development
CAROLINE MONTOJO, Dana Foundation (*as of March 2024*)

---

[1] The National Academies of Sciences, Engineering, and Medicine's forums and roundtables do not issue, review, or approve individual documents. The responsibility for the published Proceedings of a Workshop rests with the workshop rapporteurs and the institution.

JOHN NGAI, National Institute of Health's Brain Research through Advancing Innovative Neurotechnologies (BRAIN®) Initiative
GENTRY PATRICK, University of California San Diego
STEVE PAUL, Karuna Therapeutics
KATHRYN RICHMOND, Allen Institute
M. ELIZABETH ROSS, American Neurological Association
MARSIE ROSS, Harmony Biosciences
KATIE SALE, American Brain Coalition
RAYMOND SANCHEZ, Cerevel Therapeutics
TERRENCE SEJNOWSKI, Salk Institute for Biological Studies (*as of August 2023*)
SARAH SHEIKH, Takeda
SARAH SHNIDER, One Mind
DAVID SHURTLEFF, National Center for Complementary and Integrative Health
JOHN SPIRO, Simons Foundation
ALESSIO TRAVAGLIA, Foundation for the National Institutes of Health
NORA VOLKOW, National Institute on Drug Abuse
DOUG WILLIAMSON, Acadia Pharmaceuticals, Inc.
RICHARD WOYCHIK, National Institute of Environmental Health Sciences
STEVIN H. ZORN, MindImmune Therapeutics, Inc.

Forum Staff

SHEENA M. POSEY NORRIS, Director, Forum on Neuroscience and Nervous System Disorders
EVA CHILDERS, Program Officer
MAYA THIRKILL, Associate Program Officer (*as of May 2023*)
KIMBERLY OGUN, Senior Program Assistant (*as of October 2023*)
CHRISTIE BELL, Senior Finance Business Partner
CLARE STROUD, Senior Director, Board on Health Sciences Policy

Reviewers

This Proceedings of a Workshop was reviewed in draft form by individuals chosen for their diverse perspectives and technical expertise. The purpose of this independent review is to provide candid and critical comments that will assist the National Academies of Sciences, Engineering, and Medicine in making each published proceedings as sound as possible and to ensure that it meets the institutional standards for quality, objectivity, evidence, and responsiveness to the charge. The review comments and draft manuscript remain confidential to protect the integrity of the process.

We thank the following individuals for their review of this proceedings:

EVELYN POLK GREEN, Attention Deficit Disorder Association
AMELIA M. ARRIA, University of Maryland School of Public Health

Although the reviewers listed above provided many constructive comments and suggestions, they were not asked to endorse the content of the proceedings nor did they see the final draft before its release. The review of this proceedings was overseen by **BRADFORD H. GRAY,** The Urban Institute (ret.). He was responsible for making certain that an independent examination of this proceedings was carried out in accordance with standards of the National Academies and that all review comments were carefully considered. Responsibility for the final content rests entirely with the rapporteurs and the National Academies.

We also thank staff member Alexandra Beatty for reading and providing helpful comments on this manuscript.

Acknowledgments

Support from the sponsors of the Forum on Drug Discovery, Development, and Translation and the Forum on Neuroscience and Nervous System Disorders is crucial to support this and other work of the National Academies.

The National Academies staff wish to express gratitude to the Food and Drug Administration's Center for Drug Evaluation and Research for supporting this workshop in part; to the speakers whose presentations and discussions helped inform workshop discussions on the diagnosis, treatment, and drug development for adult attention-deficit/hyperactivity disorder (ADHD); to the members of the planning committee for their work in developing the workshop agenda and shaping the discussions; and to additional National Academies staff, without whom this workshop and the accounting thereof would not have been possible: Christie Bell, Lori Brenig, Samantha Chao, Robert Day, Alexandra Molina, Marguerite Romatelli, and Taryn Young.

Contents

ACRONYMS AND ABBREVIATIONS   xix

1   INTRODUCTION   1
     History of ADHD Diagnosis and Treatment, 2
     The Regulatory Landscape of Adult ADHD, 6
     Organization of the Proceedings, 7

2   ADHD DIAGNOSIS AND TREATMENT IN THE
     UNITED STATES   9
     Exploring Current ADHD Diagnosis and Treatment, 10
     Reflections on Thirty Years as an ADHD Advocate, 17

3   IMPACT OF MISDIAGNOSIS, BIAS, AND STIGMA   21
     Misdiagnosis, 22
     Stigma, Disbelief, and Inequity Surrounding Adult ADHD, 28
     Assessing Adult ADHD: Precision vs. Pragmatism, 32

4   SHARED DECISION-MAKING   37
     Adopting Measurement-Based Care, 38
     Using Shared Decision Making, 40
     Accessing Resources, 42
     Leveraging Social Media to Educate Patients, 43

5   BALANCING RISKS AND BENEFITS OF ADHD
    TREATMENT FOR ADULTS   45
    Current Pharmacologic and Nonpharmacologic Treatments, 46
    Balancing Risks and Benefits of Using ADHD Medications, 54
    Diversion and Misuse of ADHD Medication, 60

6   POTENTIAL STRATEGIES AND IMPLICATIONS FOR
    DRUG DEVELOPMENT   69
    Stimulant Drugs for ADHD, 70
    Nonstimulant Drugs for ADHD, 73
    Barriers to New Drug Development, 75
    Filling Gaps And Meeting Patients' Needs, 77

7   PUBLIC HEALTH CONSIDERATIONS AND HARM
    REDUCTION STRATEGIES   81
    A Public Health Approach to ADHD, 82
    An Integrated Treatment Model for Adult ADHD, 90
    Harm Reduction Strategies to Curb Misuse, 93
    Looking Toward the Future, 99

REFERENCES   103

APPENDIXES

A   WORKSHOP AGENDA   115

B   BIOGRAPHICAL SKETCHES OF THE WORKSHOP
    PLANNING COMMITTEE, SPEAKERS, PANELISTS, AND
    STAFF   129

Box and Figures

BOX

1-1 Workshop Statement of Task, 3

FIGURES

4-1 Tracking data from a patient undergoing ADHD treatment, comparing the HII-5 score to the PHQ-9 and GAD-7 scores, 39

5-1 Comparison of methylphenidate-based stimulants or viloxazine nonstimulant to placebo on ADHD score in adults from two randomized double-blind studies, 57
5-2 Number of stimulant prescriptions in the United States, 2012–2021, 58
5-3 Pattern of nonmedical stimulant use among U.S. individuals ages 18–50, 61
5-4 Association between stimulant treatment and substance use through adolescence into early adulthood, 64

6-1 Attention and working memory dose-response curves, 72

Acronyms and Abbreviations

ADDA	Attention Deficit Disorder Association
ADHD	attention-deficit/hyperactivity disorder
APSARD	American Professional Society of ADHD and Related Disorders
ASRS	Adult ADHD Self-Report Scale
CBT	cognitive behavioral therapy
CDC	Centers for Disease Control and Prevention
CDER	Center for Drug Evaluation and Research
CHADD	Children and Adults with ADHD
CRF	corticotropin-releasing factor
DEA	Drug Enforcement Administration
DSM-5	Diagnostic and Statistical Manual of Mental Disorders, Fifth Edition
ER	extended release
FDA	Food and Drug Administration
GAD-7	Generalized Anxiety Disorder 7-item
HII-5	Hyperactivity, Impulsivity, Inattention Symptom Rating Scale
IQ	intelligence quotient

MPH	methylphenidate
MTA	Multimodal Treatment of ADHD study
NIH	National Institutes of Health
PFC	prefrontal cortex
PHQ-9	Patient Health Questionnaire-9
SAMHSA	Substance Abuse and Mental Health Services Administration
SNRI	selective norepinephrine reuptake inhibitor
SDP	stimulant diversion prevention
SUD	substance use disorder

1

Introduction[1]

Attention-deficit/hyperactivity disorder (ADHD) is a common childhood disorder characterized by developmentally inappropriate levels of inattention, disorganization, and hyperactivity–impulsivity (APA, 2013) that can continue through adolescence and into adulthood. Studies have shown an increase over the past decade in adult ADHD diagnosis and treatment in the United States and globally (Fairman et al., 2020; Lee et al., 2021). There is evidence that adults with ADHD, including college students, may be more likely to develop a substance use disorder (SUD) and that among Medicaid-enrolled adults with ADHD, long-term use of prescription stimulants and opioids is common and increasing over time (Sepúlveda et al., 2011; Wei et al., 2018). Questions remain about the benefits and risks of prescription stimulant use for ADHD patients, particularly those with SUD. There are also concerns that the nonmedical use of prescription stimulants could lead to misuse, overdose, or toxicity.

On December 12 and 13, 2023, the Forum on Drug Discovery, Development, and Translation and the Forum on Neuroscience and Nervous System Disorders of the National Academies of Sciences, Engineering,

---

[1] This workshop was organized by an independent planning committee whose role was limited to identification of topics and speakers. This Proceedings of a Workshop was prepared by the rapporteurs as a factual summary of the presentations and discussions that took place at the workshop. Statements, recommendations, and opinions expressed are those of individual presenters and participants and are not endorsed or verified by the National Academies of Sciences, Engineering, and Medicine, and they should not be construed as reflecting any group consensus.

and Medicine convened a public workshop[2] for an array of experts in diverse fields, including clinicians, researchers, drug developers, regulators, educators, and people with lived experience to examine the diagnosis and treatment of adults with ADHD and explore the challenges and opportunities for the development of new therapeutics. Invited presentations and discussions focused on the criteria for diagnosis and treatment of adults with ADHD; risks and benefits of ADHD medication use in adult populations; nonmedical use of prescription stimulants; development of new and improved therapeutics; and potential strategies for assessing the risks and benefits of treatment that support the public health goal of safely and effectively treating adults with ADHD (see Box 1-1).

HISTORY OF ADHD DIAGNOSIS AND TREATMENT

Craig Surman, director of the Clinical and Research Program in Adult ADHD at Massachusetts General Hospital and associate professor of psychiatry at Harvard Medical School, provided a brief overview of the history of ADHD diagnosis and treatment. Since it was described in the early 1900s, what is now called ADHD has primarily been considered a disease of children. For almost a century, doctors did not meaningfully consider what happens to these children when they grow up. Nonetheless, half of all children diagnosed with ADHD continue to experience symptoms in adulthood, while others do not receive a diagnosis until they are grown (Faraone et al., 2024). ADHD "appears to be an exacerbator," said Surman; "whatever other challenges an individual faces, it amplifies." Although environment alone does not create ADHD, inequity heightens its affects. Children with socioeconomic disadvantage often have higher rates of diagnosis and experience the greatest suffering from ADHD (Faraone et al., 2024).

ADHD affects 4 percent of adults in the United States (ADDA, 2022), said Ann Childress, president of the Center for Psychiatry and Behavioral Medicine, Inc., and the American Professional Society of ADHD and Related Disorders (APSARD). ADHD presents differently in adults than in children, but its effects are no less harmful in adults than children (ADDA, 2022). The disorder disrupts relationships, careers, physical health, mental health, and even lifespan, added Surman. ADHD may put individuals at increased risk of developing a substance use disorder (FDA and DEA, 2023). However, the lack of research on adult ADHD has led to major gaps in knowledge and contributed to the widespread misdiagnosis and mis-

---

[2] A recording of the full workshop can be found on the event's webpage, https://www.nationalacademies.org/event/40683_12-2023_adult-attention-deficit-hyperactivity-disorder-drug-development-diagnosis-and-treatment-a-workshop (accessed April 24, 2024).

BOX 1-1
Workshop Statement of Task

A planning committee of the National Academies of Sciences, Engineering, and Medicine will organize a public workshop that will provide an opportunity for professionals who typically diagnose attention-deficit/hyperactivity disorder (ADHD) (e.g., physicians, psychologists, social workers, nurse practitioners, and other licensed counselors or therapists), drug developers, researchers, regulators, patients, and other stakeholders to examine the diagnosis and treatment of adults with ADHD and explore the challenges and opportunities for the development of new therapeutics. The public workshop will feature invited presentations and discussions to:

- Discuss the criteria for diagnosis and treatment of adults with ADHD, taking into consideration health disparities and perspectives of people with lived experience;
- Consider what is known and unknown about the risks and benefits of ADHD medication use in adult populations;
- Share perspectives on the causes, perceptions, consequences, and health equity implications of nonmedical use of prescription stimulants, including misuse potential, overdosage, and toxicity;
- Explore challenges and opportunities for the development of new and improved therapeutics for the treatment of ADHD; and
- Consider potential strategies for assessing the risks and benefits of ADHD medication treatment in adult populations, including the intersection with opioid use, that support the public health goal of safely and effectively treating adults with ADHD.

The planning committee will organize the workshop, develop the agenda, select and invite speakers and discussants, and moderate or identify moderators for the discussions. A proceedings of the presentations and discussions at the workshop will be prepared by a designated rapporteur in accordance with institutional guidelines.

---

treatment of this population (Ramos-Quiroga et al., 2014). Furthermore, tightened restrictions on stimulant medications in the United States and a recent shortage of these drugs, combined with a significant increase in the diagnosis and treatment of adult ADHD over the past decade (FDA and DEA, 2023), have highlighted the unmet needs of adult ADHD patients and the shortcomings of the current treatment landscape.

ADHD is Defined by Behavior

Historically, ADHD has been defined based on behavior, and overwhelmingly in children, said Surman. Attributing the cause to brain damage, early twentieth-century constructs of ADHD were lumped together with learning disabilities, impulsivity with hyperkinesis, and short attention span. By the 1930s, ADHD symptoms evolved into "minimal brain dysfunction." The diagnosis became known as hyperactive child syndrome in the 1960s, with a focus on motor symptoms (Lange et al., 2010). Attentional problems did not enter the diagnostic criteria until 1980, which means that many of today's adults with ADHD might have been diagnosed differently as children, noted Surman. The late 1980s and 1990s marked important milestones for individuals with ADHD, with the founding of patient advocacy organizations,[3] the consequent allocation of resources to support the education of affected children, and a National Institutes of Health (NIH) consensus conference supporting the validity of the Diagnostic and Statistical Manual of Mental Disorders definition of ADHD (NIH, 1998), said Surman.

Seven major longitudinal studies conducted in North America between 1961 and 1999 followed individuals for up to 33 years, informing the understanding that ADHD could apply to adults (Cherkasova et al., 2022). These studies showed that about half of children with ADHD continue to have the full condition into adulthood, said Surman. However, diagnosis of ADHD in adults is complicated by high rates of concurrent mental health and neurological conditions, masking of obvious impairment by environmental or personal compensatory efforts, as well as lack of awareness of or access to clinical care for ADHD.

The current diagnosis for ADHD found in the Fifth Edition of the Diagnostic and Statistical Manual of Mental Disorders (DSM-5) relies entirely on behavior, as most individuals with ADHD do not differ significantly from individuals without ADHD in terms of brain imaging or functional tests, said Surman. Because two or more roles or areas of functions must be impaired to obtain a diagnosis of ADHD and because verification of the required onset of symptoms by the age of 12 is challenging, a population of "diagnostic orphans" may experience significant impairment but nonetheless fail to qualify as having ADHD, he said. Since the 1990s, influential scholarship has highlighted the role of emotional discontrol as a core feature of ADHD (Wender, 1995), but the current DSM-5 ADHD diagnostic criteria, solidified in 2013, still do not include that feature, said Surman.

---

[3] Two patient advocacy groups represented among the participants were Children and Adults with Attention-Deficit/Hyperactivity Disorder, https://chadd.org, and the Attention Deficit Disorder Association, https://add.org (both accessed March 2, 2024).

Genetic and Environmental Risk Factors

Based on family and twin studies (Asherson and Gurling, 2011; Larsson et al., 2014), 70 percent of ADHD is thought to be due to genetic inheritance, said Surman. However, it not explained by any single gene; instead, multiple genes seem to be responsible (Pujol-Gualdo et al., 2021). Surman explained that many types of environmental risks are also correlated with ADHD, including premature birth, low socioeconomic support, fetal toxicity, and parental cigarette smoking (Bernardina Dalla et al., 2022; Crump et al., 2023; Kim et al., 2020; Russell et al., 2014).

Slower maturation of the prefrontal cortex (PFC) has been observed in some individuals with ADHD (Shaw et al., 2007), consistent with observations of delayed maturity in self-regulatory abilities in individuals with ADHD, said Surman. Furthermore, he continued, those with and without ADHD perform differently on neuropsychological tasks, including tests of working memory, attention, and other executive functions (Arrondo et al., 2024; Leib et al., 2021). However, many people who meet the full DSM-5 criteria for ADHD show no difference in brain imaging or test-based performance. Surman said this is not surprising, considering that the DSM-5 diagnosis relies entirely on behavioral symptoms and functional impairment, which are largely descriptive criteria (Leffa et al., 2022).

Overview of ADHD Treatment

"The history of ADHD treatment is one of opportunistic use of agents that were developed a long time ago," said Surman (Connolly et al., 2015). The positive effects of using amphetamines in children with ADHD were first reported in 1937. Methylphenidate (MPH) was synthesized a decade later, and now there are multiple formulations of both drugs, he said. These stimulants boost levels of dopamine and norepinephrine by blocking their reuptake at the synapse and, in the case of amphetamines, by increasing dopamine and norepinephrine release. Surman explained that the effects of these drugs vary from person to person, and they can change with habituation. Effects of ADHD drugs are broad and can impact energy, alertness, and the sympathetic nervous system, including the cardiovascular system. Rapid absorption can lead to euphoric effects, said Surman.

Stimulants can be habit-forming, said Surman. He noted that the newer, longer-release formulations of methylphenidate and amphetamine, which have different patterns of absorption and longer-lasting effects than the initial formulations, may be less appealing for diversion and misuse (Groom and Cortese, 2022). Four nonstimulant drugs—atomoxetine, clonidine extended release (ER), guanfacine ER, and viloxazine—are currently approved by the U.S. Food and Drug Administration (FDA) for treating ADHD (FDA, 2023b). Of these, only atomoxetine and viloxazine ER are approved for use in adults. However, it is not uncommon for guanfacine ER and clonidine ER, which are approved for children and adolescents but not adults, to be used off-label for adults (Iwanami et al., 2020). Each of these is thought to modulate norepinephrine more than dopamine (CHADD, 2023), said Surman.

THE REGULATORY LANDSCAPE OF ADULT ADHD

Marta Sokolowska, deputy center director for Substance Use and Behavioral Health at the Center for Drug Evaluation and Research (CDER) at the FDA, provided a brief overview of the regulatory landscape and the agency's actions taken in response to a significant spike in adult ADHD prescriptions, the rise in telemedicine, and the concern regarding nonmedical and misuse of prescription stimulants. Robert Califf, Commissioner of the FDA, highlighted the conflicting needs that make ADHD treatment so complicated, namely, providing effective treatment to adults with ADHD while curbing misuse of stimulant medications. Medications for ADHD have clear short-term and long-term benefits for both children and adults, said Califf. "Untreated ADHD has a range of adverse consequences," he said, and treatment with stimulants results in better academic performance and fewer injuries, SUDs, and criminal acts. While acknowledging the tremendous importance of treating ADHD, Califf noted that stimulants are Schedule II medications with significant potential for abuse and dependence. He referenced the 2022 National Survey on Drug Use and Health, which found that 800,000 people began misusing prescription stimulants in 2022, and 1.8 million had a prescription stimulant use disorder, with the highest rates among young adults aged 18 to 25 (SAMHSA, 2023). Califf emphasized the need for patients and providers to "find the right balance" between enabling access to medication for those who would benefit from treatment and minimizing exposure to medications for those who would not benefit.

This workshop, said Califf, is critical for making progress on key issues, including questions about how ADHD is currently diagnosed in adults, the validity of diagnostic tools, how to increase the use of evidence-based tools for diagnosis, and how to understand the balance of long-term safety and effectiveness of current treatments. Califf asked participants to consider what data are needed to address questions about overtreatment, inappropriate prescribing, and stimulant misuse. Finally, he asked workshop participants to consider what sort of professional and clinical framework would optimize appropriate diagnosis and treatment and minimize inappropriate treatment.

ORGANIZATION OF THE PROCEEDINGS

This Proceedings of a Workshop summarizes the presentations and discussions that took place during the public workshop held on December 12 and 13, 2023. Chapter 2 presents a brief overview of ADHD diagnosis and treatment in the United States, from the lack of guidelines for diagnosis and treatment to medication misuse and diversion. Participants considered the types and extent of stimulant misuse, while panelists with ADHD recounted their experiences seeking treatment and managing unmedicated ADHD during the drug shortage. Chapter 3 discusses misdiagnosis, bias, and stigma and their effects on patient care. Chapter 4 explores shared decision making between patients and their providers. Chapter 5 considers the risks and benefits of different ways to treat adult ADHD from both the patient and provider perspective. Chapters 6 discusses implications for drug development. Finally, the proceedings concludes in Chapter 7 with public health considerations and harm reduction strategies. Each chapter includes the reflections and perspectives of those living with adult ADHD. The workshop agenda can be found in Appendix A and biographical sketches of the workshop planning committee members, speakers, and panelists in Appendix B.

2

ADHD Diagnosis and Treatment in the United States

Highlights of Key Points Made by Individual Speakers*

- ADHD among adults in the United States is a common mental health condition. The condition impairs social, academic, and occupational functioning. The burden of ADHD includes lower earnings, lower academic achievement, more car crashes, and an increased risk of death compared to unaffected peers. (Childress)
- Most adults living with ADHD have at least one comorbid psychiatric disorder and the spectrum of symptoms and co-morbidities is different for men and women. This makes diagnosis in adults complex, and many practitioners may lack adequate knowledge about how to properly diagnose and treat adults with ADHD. (Childress, Sibley)
- ADHD looks very different in adults compared to children, yet diagnostic tools for adults still rely on symptoms as presented in children. (Higgins, Sibley)
- Accurately diagnosing ADHD in adults requires integrating information from across multiple sources and can take more time than the average office visit. (Higgins, Sibley)
- "Adults don't need to be told what to do or what's wrong with them. They need the tools and strategies to implement those tools, and they need knowledge and community sup-

---

port. They need to know all the ways they can manage their ADHD without bias." (Green)

*This list is the rapporteurs' summary of points made by the individual speakers identified, and the statements have not been endorsed or verified by the National Academies of Sciences, Engineering, and Medicine. They are not intended to reflect a consensus among workshop participants.

The workshop began with an overview of how ADHD in adults is diagnosed and the various treatment options available to them. Presentations and panel discussions focused on the criteria and available tools for diagnosis of ADHD in adults; challenges to appropriate diagnosis of ADHD for different adult populations; and the implications of treatment options.

EXPLORING CURRENT ADHD DIAGNOSIS AND TREATMENT

Adult ADHD: Definition, Diagnosis, and Prevalence

ADHD is characterized by "impairing levels of inattention, disorganization, and/or hyperactivity-impulsivity," said Childress (APA, 2013). To qualify as ADHD, Childress explained that impairment must begin before age 12, it must interfere with functioning or development, and other conditions must be ruled out. ADHD often continues into adulthood, where it impairs social, academic, and occupational functioning. Though not included in the clinical definition, emotional dysregulation or impulsivity is another hallmark of ADHD, she said (Childress, 2023).

The prevalence of ADHD among adults (ages 18 to 55), in the United States is estimated at 4.4 percent (Kessler, 2006), making it one of the most prevalent mental health disorders, said Surman. A prevalence of 4.4 percent places ADHD as the third most prevalent mental health conditions U.S. adults experience, behind generalized anxiety and major depression, respectively (NAMI, 2023). Childress expanded that in adults overall, ADHD is slightly more prevalent in men than women and continues to be seen in adults as they age, with some studies indicating a 2.8 percent prevenance among adults ages 60 and older (Michielsen et al., 2012; Solberg et al., 2018). Overall, prevalence is lower in African Americans, Native Americans, Pacific Islanders, and Asian Americans compared to Whites (Chung et al., 2019), but Childress acknowledged that those populations are vastly underrepresented. She continued to explain that the burden carried by those with ADHD includes lower earnings, lower academic achievement, more car crashes, and an increased risk of death when compared to unaffected peers (Mustonen et al., 2023). ADHD alone increases the risk of death 1.5-fold. When combined with one comorbid condition like depression or anxiety, the risk increases fourfold. Two comorbid conditions along with ADHD increase the risk of death by a factor of eight; three comorbid conditions increase the risk by a factor of 15; and four comorbid conditions increase it by a factor of 29 (Solberg et al., 2018).

On a societal level, adult ADHD costs the United States in excess of $100 billion annually, said Surman. Furthermore, "ADHD leaves a trail of challenges far beyond individuals themselves," continued Surman, causing damage within families, educational settings, the workplace, and society at large (Schein et al., 2022). As many as a quarter of individuals in the criminal legal system could meet diagnostic criteria for ADHD, he noted.

Tools for Diagnosing ADHD in Adults

Diagnosing ADHD correctly requires a thorough clinical history, which takes time to collect, said Childress. The clinical interview should inquire about symptoms, impairments, and comorbid conditions. Given the strong heritable nature of ADHD, a thorough family history will probably identify an affected relative, she added. It is important to look for other medical conditions that might cause ADHD-like symptoms and for conditions that might complicate treatment, such as cardiac issues. The interview includes use of rating scales, which can be either patient reported or clinician administered. Childress recommended the Adult ADHD Self-Report Scale (ASRS-v1.1),[1] which scores the 18 criteria specified in DSM-5 and can be completed in about five minutes. Childress referenced various other diagnostic tools typically used in clinical trials, including the Adult ADHD Clinical Diagnostic Scale (Adler et al., 2017) and the Adult ADHD Investigator Symptom Rating Scale (Spencer et al., 2010). She highlighted that while the scales rate executive function, quality of life, and impairment, they are not practical for general use due to their time requirement.

Several participants emphasized the need for short diagnostic questionnaires that could be completed quickly. This is particularly necessary for teachers, who are typically the first to detect ADHD in children, said Napoleon Higgins, president and chief executive officer of Bay Pointe Behavioral Health. "As a former teacher," he said, "please do not hand me a scale that has 100 questions [while] I am working . . . with 20 other

---

[1] Available at https://www.apaservices.org/practice/reimbursement/health-registry/self-reporting-sympton-scale.pdf (accessed March 14, 2024).

kids. . . . The shorter the questionnaire, the more likely . . . it [will be] accurate."

Comorbidities and Gender Differences

More than 70 percent of adults with ADHD have at least one comorbid psychiatric disorder, said Childress (Pehlivanidis et al., 2020). Approximately 55 percent of adults with ADHD have depressive disorders, 47 percent have anxiety disorders, 41 percent have SUDs, and 35 percent have bipolar disorder. Childress stressed the importance of screening for these comorbidities in clinical practice, indicating she uses for this purpose the Mini-International Neuropsychiatric Interview (Sheehan et al., 1998), which "can get through the entire DSM in 15 to 30 minutes."

Among adults with ADHD, the spectrum of symptoms and comorbidities varies based on gender, said Childress (Young et al., 2020). Men have more externalizing problems like antisocial behaviors, while women are more likely to have emotional problems, anxiety, depression, and borderline personality traits. Women with ADHD are also at a higher risk for severe mental illness, such as schizophrenia (Young et al., 2020). Symptoms of ADHD may be less overt in women, leading to a delay in diagnosis, she said. Childress has seen many adult women patients who had been diagnosed with anxiety and treatment-resistant depression that turned out to be driven by ADHD. "When the ADHD was treated," she said, "the depression got better."

Choosing ADHD Treatments

All ADHD drugs have possible adverse physical, mental, and cardio-vascular effects, said Surman. However, of the many versions of stimulants currently on the market, only six of the long-acting formulations include data generated from adult experiences on the label. There are few clinical studies that compare one drug to another, so "clinicians need to draw . . . largely from their own experience" when choosing which drugs to prescribe, he said.

Comparisons between nonstimulants and stimulants are also complicated by several other factors, including differences in dosing between the two types of medication. Surman said that drug labels tend to indicate higher effects for stimulants than nonstimulants, which is likely one reason nonstimulant medications are not as commonly prescribed for ADHD in the United States. Many adults take multiple drugs to treat other conditions in addition to ADHD, creating issues of polypharmacy, he noted. Study populations exclude many individuals who have co-occurring conditions that affect their mental health.

The only way to understand the unintended long-term health effects of treatments is to study users for long time periods—longer than controlled clinical studies allow, said Surman. For this reason, he emphasized the "incredible importance" of the system of postmarket surveillance that allows patients to be followed indefinitely. The large longitudinal datasets that have been collected by countries with centralized health records, such as Sweden and Denmark (Schmidt et al., 2015; Swedish National Board of Health and Welfare, 2019), are also proving valuable, he said.

Medication is not the only effective treatment for ADHD, noted Surman. Cognitive behavioral therapy (CBT) has been shown to work well when combined with medication (Lopez et al., 2018). While ADHD is a disability covered by the Rehabilitation Act of 1973[2] and the Americans with Disabilities Act of 1990,[3] accommodations are not treatments, Surman noted. However, he said, an environment of accommodation can make a real difference in the lives of people with ADHD. While most accommodation has occurred in educational settings, workplaces are now learning how to implement practices that accommodate neurodiversity, he added.

A Snapshot of Adult ADHD Care in the United States

Childress shared early results of a survey she and colleagues at Medscape conducted during the early stages of the ongoing 2022 stimulant shortage to understand how clinicians were addressing adult ADHD during this time. The survey began in November 2023 and included health care providers and patients (Childress, 2023). Childress presented data from the first three weeks of the clinician survey. The survey questioned attitudes, skills, competence, barriers to diagnosis, and the burden of treatment as perceived by physicians and nurse practitioners. On questions of adult ADHD prevalence, risk factors, comorbidities, and impact, only 45 percent answered questions correctly, said Childress. Only 41 percent correctly identified the diagnostic criteria and knew about screening tools and underdiagnosis. Although 71 percent correctly answered questions about treatment outcomes, only 49 percent knew about all the available treatments. In short, "There is a huge lack of knowledge . . . [even though] these are people that are treating ADHD," she said.

Regarding the types of drugs being prescribed, 84 percent of the clinicians reported prescribing short-acting stimulants, and less than half of these switched to prescribing nonstimulants in the wake of the stimulant shortage (Childress, 2023). In many cases, insurance carriers pushed pro-

---

[2] Rehabilitation Act of 1973, Section 504, Public Law 112, 93rd Cong. (September 26, 1973).
[3] Americans with Disabilities Act of 1990, Public Law 336, 101st Cong. (July 26, 1990).

viders to prescribe short-acting stimulants by requiring prior authorization for nonstimulants or refusing them altogether, said Childress.

In Childress's survey of patients with ADHD, individuals were asked
about the burden of illness and barriers to treatment. More than half
reported multiple quality-of-life issues that were negatively impacted by
ADHD, including memory or cognition, work or school, getting to places
on time, sleep, finances, and relationships. Sixty-eight percent had also
been diagnosed with an anxiety disorder and 49 percent with depression. Nonetheless, only half of the respondents were currently undergoing treatment for their ADHD. Half of those in treatment were receiving
long-acting stimulants, 37 percent were on short-acting stimulants, and
21 percent received nonstimulant medicine. Half were in counseling or
therapy. Only 28 percent of those on stimulants were completely satisfied with their care. Medicine shortages were reported by 41 percent of
patients overall. The single most important consideration for patients
when choosing a treatment for ADHD was cost. When asked to name the
top barriers affecting their ability to get treated for ADHD, patients cited
difficulties obtaining a controlled medicine; the drug being out of stock;
the drug being too expensive (or not covered by insurance); and troubles
dealing with the health care system.

Summarizing her results, Childress said that ADHD is common and
its diagnosis in adults is complex, but it can be effectively treated. However, many practitioners lack knowledge about adult ADHD. Half of
patients are not getting treatment, and the cost of medication and insurance coverage are a huge barrier to care.

Lara Robinson, behavioral scientist for the National Center on Birth
Defects and Developmental Disabilities at the Centers for Disease Control
and Prevention (CDC), presented preliminary results from the CDC's Fall
2023 Porter Novelli DocStyles Survey,[4] which asked providers of ADHD
care for both adults and children about ADHD identification, treatment,
referral, knowledge, and resources. Approximately 1,500 practitioners
were surveyed, with half of child providers and two-thirds of adult providers reporting inadequate training in ADHD, said Robinson.

Lack of Guidelines for Diagnosis and Treatment
of Adult ADHD in the United States

"One of the leading challenges in finding the right balance around the
diagnosis and treatment of ADHD is that there are currently no United
States guidelines for diagnosing and treating adults with ADHD," said
Califf, calling the establishment of guidelines "a necessary step in advanc-

---

[4] Available at https://styles.porternovelli.com/docstyles/ (accessed April 26, 2024).

ing the quality of care." The United Kingdom, Canada, the European Union, and Australia have published adult ADHD practice guidelines (Alliance, 2020; Kooij et al., 2010; May et al., 2023; NICE, 2018), noted both Childress and David Goodman, assistant professor of psychiatry and behavioral sciences at Johns Hopkins University School of Medicine. "The U.S. is the only major developed country without either national or regional guidelines on [adult] ADHD diagnosis," said Margaret Sibley, professor of psychiatry and behavioral sciences at the University of Washington School of Medicine. Diagnosis of ADHD in adults still relies on symptoms as presented in children, reflecting a dearth of data on how the disease plays out in adults, she added.

An APSARD task force is performing the critical task of "aggregating our communal empirical, clinical and experiential knowledge" to develop national guidelines for diagnosing and treating adult ADHD, said Sibley. Working with the guidelines developed by APSARD, Children and Adults with ADHD (CHADD) will develop professional toolkits tailored to specific medical specialties as well as parents and caretakers, noted Goodman along with Russell Ramsay, cofounder and former codirector of the Adult ADHD Treatment and Research Program at the University of Pennsylvania, and Mary Solanto, professor of pediatrics and psychiatry at the Zucker School of Medicine at Hofstra-Northwell.

Califf urged that the process of developing the guidelines be adequate to address concerns of bias or conflict of interest. He cautioned that guidelines can be "treacherous" when clinical evidence is inadequate. "We lack fundamental information on who should be treated, disparities in diagnosis, and assessments of clinical practice that would allow us to make rational decisions about how to approach supply and demand," he said, suggesting that clinical guidelines distinguish between recommendations based on high-quality evidence and those based solely on expert opinion. Goodman described the "tediousness and difficulty [and] rigor" that is going into development of the guidelines (Goodman, 2023; Goodman and Mattingly, 2023).

Key questions about ADHD symptoms can be addressed through well-funded and thoughtfully designed studies, said Sibley. However, even though adults make up a majority of the U.S. population with ADHD (Cortese et al., 2023; Song et al., 2021), active NIH research spending on ADHD in adults in 2023 was "just a sliver" of what was spent on ADHD research overall and less than 1 percent of the $650 million spent on depression research, she added. ADHD is the second most prevalent psychiatric disorder, Goodman pointed out and called the lack of funding for research on adults with ADHD "appalling."

Diagnostic tools need to be improved to be "more efficient and more accurate," said Sibley, but this is difficult without crucial data. "We have very little collective knowledge of what adult ADHD looks like, whether it can be transient, environmentally determined, gender specific, hormonally influenced, secondary to other problems, or late onset," she said. Further complicating efforts at diagnosis, she added, "we do not have language to describe ADHD-like symptoms that are not ADHD."

Solving the dilemma of who should be treated for ADHD, and how, will require research that seeks to answer fundamental questions about the epidemiology of ADHD and the risk-benefit balance of treatment in diverse patient populations, said Califf. While research "has not shown a causative progression from the use of prescription stimulants to the use of illegal stimulants . . . absence of evidence is not the same as evidence of absence," said Califf, particularly in light of the recent increase in prescription stimulant use and the widespread availability of amphetamines outside prescription channels. Citing this and other questions regarding the use of stimulants to treat ADHD in adults, Califf committed himself to working with colleagues across the Department of Health and Human Services "to explore these topics in the detail that they deserve."

Concerns Regarding Misuse, Abuse, and Diversion of Prescription Stimulants

Recognizing that many FDA-approved drugs to treat adult ADHD are stimulants, concerns about misuse of ADHD drugs have led to strict controls on access, and these controls contributed to a recent, nationwide shortage of prescription medication for ADHD (FDA, 2023a; Scott, 2023; Wolkoff Wachsman, 2023). Workshop participants considered the types and extent of stimulant misuse, while panelists with ADHD recounted their experiences seeking treatment and managing unmedicated ADHD during the drug shortage.

Misuse, abuse, and diversion of prescription stimulants constituted one of the focal points of this workshop. Surman offered the following definitions for these terms within the context of the workshop:

- *Misuse* is improper or unhealthy use of a prescription drug, including without a prescription of one's own or in a way other than prescribed, such as in greater amounts, more often, or for a longer period than prescribed (SAMHSA, 2021);
- *Abuse* is the misuse of a drug (prescription, illicit, psychoactive substance, or alcohol) to get high or inflect self-harm (FDA, 2017; SAMHSA, 2005); and
- *Diversion* is when a drug is directed outside of prescribed channels, for example, to a different marketplace or shared between individuals (CMS, 2016).

The literature on misuse, abuse, and diversion of medication by adults with ADHD centers around college-age students, said Surman, where medication misuse happens with a 10 to 20 percent prevalence (Benson et al., 2015). In 2015 the Substance Abuse and Mental Health Services Administration (SAMHSA) reported a 10 percent lifetime misuse of stimulants, with peak occurrence at age 21 (Hughes, 2016). Most prescription stimulant diversion occurred between friends. Some individuals with ADHD may seek medications outside the regulated marketplace, where fake pills may contain dangerous chemicals such as methamphetamine and fentanyl, noted Surman.

REFLECTIONS ON THIRTY YEARS AS AN ADHD ADVOCATE

Evelyn Polk Green is the immediate past president the Attention Deficit Disorder Association (ADDA), the past president of CHADD, an adult with ADHD, and the mother of two adult sons with ADHD. Many of the items discussed at this workshop were being talked about 30 years ago, she said, noting that while some things have improved, many still have not.

Green was a "poster child" for undiagnosed ADHD until adulthood. As a child with a supportive family, she did well in school and attended Duke University on a full scholarship. Away from her supportive home environment, everything "literally fell apart around my ears." After Green married and had her first child, she mustered the strength to earn three degrees, and then was diagnosed with ADHD shortly after her youngest son was diagnosed. Green started the first urban CHADD chapter, in Chicago, after a suburban parent explained to her that "kids in the city don't have ADHD. They [have] emotional and behavioral disturbances." Before long, Green had joined the CHADD national board and become president.

Until Green started treating her ADHD with medication, she said, "I had no idea how good life could be." But things fell apart again at perimenopause and menopause. Green told her story to illustrate that, for an adult with ADHD, life has "ups and downs and ins and outs. I never know when I wake up what life is going to be . . . and even when it looks good on the outside, some of us are really good at masking. Know that as you work with your adult clients and patients."

Green, who is Black, discovered early "that the only way things were going to be changed was if we told our story." But the stigma and the shame around ADHD reduce people's willingness to do so, especially people from Black and Brown communities, she explained. Over her three decades in advocacy, Green has spoken with thousands of adults with ADHD. She remains "disappointed, maybe even a little disgusted," that "the real impact of untreated ADHD on both the individual and society as a whole" is still not taken as seriously as it should be. "Folks don't get the trauma that's involved, the heartache, the shame, the stigma . . . and how much we need you to support us to get through that."

Treating Adult Patients as Partners

"Sometimes it feels like adults with ADHD are treated the way children with ADHD are treated by the clinicians and the researchers . . . like we can't figure it out for ourselves, like we don't need to be partners in decisions about our lives and treatment," Green said. Adults with ADHD should be empowered and engaged as partners in their own treatment or that treatment will never succeed, she said. "Adults don't need to be told what to do or what's wrong with them. They need the tools and strategies to implement those tools, and they need knowledge and community support. They need to know all the ways they can manage their ADHD without bias," she said. Green cited an adage from the disability movement, "Nothing about us without us," and remarked that this workshop was the first time that adults living with ADHD had been asked for their opinions in a national scientific forum.

Green noted the important roles played by both CHADD and ADDA, the two leading organizations that advocate for people with ADHD. CHADD is vital, she said, but ADDA deals exclusively with adults, and "you need to take advantage of what both of them have to offer." ADDA was started "because nobody else was giving adults with ADHD the respect and information that they needed." ADDA does not hear enough from the research community, she continued. "You don't ask enough questions," she said. While it is important to ensure that CHADD works with the professional organizations on developing guidelines, "let's also make sure that we give the adults access to those tools and guidelines, so they know what questions to ask when they go in . . . so they make those decisions." Furthermore, "I heard a thousand times about the diversity we need," in ADHD research, she added. "Most of the respondents were White, because that's where you went to ask the questions." She noted that ADDA has support groups for lesbian, gay, bisexual, transgender and queer persons, Black people, Asian people, and others. "We just need to ask the right questions and ask the right people," she said.

There is one big lesson to be learned from pediatric ADHD treatment, said Green. "Who treats pediatric ADHD? Pediatricians." In contrast, she said, "family practitioners, [primary care physicians], general practitioners are not the ones treating adult ADHD. . . . Something is wrong," and it is a reason why adults do not get diagnosed.

Adult ADHD Remains a "Black Hole"

Green related some of the questions she encounters around adult ADHD. She is frequently asked whether it is real, "which is very sad. . . . Let me give you a day out of my life, and I'll show you just how real it is." Adults with ADHD "want to know what they can do to help themselves and where they can get support and find community." Educators want to know what kind of accommodations they can make to help kids with ADHD succeed. Green noted that, like many clinicians, teachers receive no training on ADHD or guidance on what to do "when those kids land in front of them . . . and there's at least one in every classroom."

Far too often, said Green, "people still think of ADHD as a disorder of little hyperactive White boys." Diagnosis of adults with ADHD remains "a big black hole for a lot of folks, and we need more answers," she added.

Tension Between Stimulant Misuse and Patient Access to Care

Concerns about SUD and misuse can dominate the discussion of adult ADHD, said Green. "It's prevalent to the point that all the attention is focused there, instead of on the everyday adult with ADHD that's not trying to abuse [or divert] their Adderall. . . . Let's put the attention where it needs to be," she advised. "We talk a lot about misuse, but I want to remind you that misuse can also be caused by giving the wrong person the wrong medication."

Diversion was such a concern when Green's son went to college that he insisted on switching to a nonstimulant, but that medication adversely impacted his academic performance, she said. "None of us in the advocacy community want [diversion], because it reflects badly on us . . . but we need to have balance and not always assume the worst. . . . It's almost like an assumption that adults with ADHD are going to misuse, [that] they all want to be addicts," she said. In response to providers' fears of a patient faking ADHD, Green countered, "it's really hard to fake impairment." Instead of relying on a checklist of what ADHD supposedly looks like, she said, "clinicians need to ask the right questions. . . . How many car accidents have you had? How many people have you run over? How many times have you lost your keys, and in what situations?"

Unmet Needs: Training and Community Engagement

The single most important change needed to improve care for adults with ADHD is training doctors and psychologists, said Green. When faced with the argument that "everybody thinks their [discipline] is the most important and wants to add more training" for physicians and nurse practitioners in the field, she said, "I get that, nobody really has time. But we need to make time, because it's important." Furthermore, adult ADHD should be covered in the initial training of providers, not just as continuing education. Indeed, she added, "if we just train people to be more empathetic, to ask the right questions, that would make a huge difference to ADHD and all kinds of other issues."

Green cited additional "30-year issues that are still there." High on this list is the need to train "more clinicians that look like us, and sound like us, and understand us." Another persistent problem is the lack of representation of minorities in clinical trials, which creates an inequitable treatment landscape, Green said. She recounted "parents who said to me, 'I don't care what they say about that medication being safe, they didn't try it out on my kid, they didn't try it out on Black kids'. . . . So we have to look at how we're recruiting people . . . and what we can do differently to make sure that we are being inclusive."

Lastly, Green noted that "stigma is still a thing . . . specifically for Black and Brown families. It's not just the external stigma, it's the internal family stigma that you have to deal with. It's so complicated." Green continues to advocate, she said, because "the only way that we can stop stigma is for people to stand up and talk about their experiences . . . and to share that information with others. It's not an easy thing to do, it's not. But that I think is the only way that we're going to overcome it."

3

Impact of Misdiagnosis, Bias, and Stigma

Highlights of Key Points Made by Individual Speakers*

- Clinicians not adequately trained to diagnose and treat ADHD in adults may lead to underdiagnosis and suboptimal treatment. (Goodman, Mahome, Olfson)
- ADHD is more challenging to diagnose in adults than in children because symptoms in adults are heterogeneous, many adults test false positive on screening tests, and clinicians disagree on the threshold of symptoms needed for a diagnosis. Comorbidities, trauma, adversity, and substance use can also complicate the diagnosis of ADHD in adults. (Higgins, Lee, Sibley, Surman, Walker)
- Underdiagnosis of ADHD in disadvantaged groups exacerbates health inequities. Access to appropriate ADHD diagnosis is subject to many biases related to race, gender, age, employment, and socioeconomic status. (El-Sabawi, Goodman, Gordon, Higgins, Mahome, Rosier, Schatz)
- Black and Brown men are frequently misdiagnosed with oppositional defiant or conduct disorders, and women across races and ethnicities are more likely to be diagnosed with anxiety and depression. (Higgins, Goodman)
- A diagnosis of ADHD carries considerable stigma, particularly among racial and ethnic minorities. Adults may not be diagnosed until they become unable to manage their personal

---

or professional obligations, which may be interpreted as fail-
ing or a character flaw, leading to feelings of shame. (Baker,
Goodman, Gordon, Higgins, Rosier)

- Practitioners worrying about patients' faking it further stigma-
tizes mental health. Impairment cannot be faked. (Farchione,
Mahome, Walker)

*This list is the rapporteurs' summary of points made by the
individual speakers identified, and the statements have not been
endorsed or verified by the National Academies of Sciences,
Engineering, and Medicine. They are not intended to reflect a
consensus among workshop participants.

"ADHD has a childhood face," said Higgins, with many of the diagnostic criteria are based on children. ADHD is easy to pick up in a ram-
bunctious young boy, but affected adults do not typically run around the
workplace and climb on desks. Instead, he said, ADHD is likely to play
out in adults as an executive function issue that rears its head in college
or later in adult life, when individuals have to juggle family and career
obligations. "Life gets faster and it catches up with you. . . . [This] is where
I see a lot of the misdiagnosis," he said.

"The lived experiences of individuals with ADHD are suggesting a
range of adult expressions of ADHD that are yet to be empirically con-
firmed as core features of the disorder," Sibley said. In the United States,
there are twice as many adults with ADHD as children with ADHD
(IQVIA, 2023), noted David Baker, former pharmaceutical executive and
current board member for Edge Foundation. Nonetheless, underdiagnosis
among adults was consistently raised by panelists with lived experience.
"It's not at all uncommon for adults to be diagnosed after their children,"
said Duane Gordon, president of ADDA, who first sought care after his
daughter was diagnosed with ADHD. Clinicians in attendance, including
Childress, mentioned that mothers often ask them for their own evaluation after one of their children have been diagnosed.

MISDIAGNOSIS

ADHD is more challenging to diagnose in adults than in children, and
there are several reasons for this, Sibley said. First, most attention problems are not related to ADHD. Concentration difficulties are the second
most common symptom listed for conditions within the entire DSM-5.
Adults have decades of accumulated illnesses, injuries, traumas, anxieties,

sleep problems, and behaviors that can be confused with ADHD, and all of these can also be comorbid with ADHD. Indeed, 20 to 30 percent of all adults report elevated ADHD-like symptoms on screening tests at some point in their life, and nearly 90 percent of these are false positives (Chamberlain et al., 2021; Sibley et al., 2018), she said.

Second, clinicians may be unsure when symptoms are severe enough for a diagnosis of ADHD, said Sibley. ADHD is a polygenic disorder that is influenced by the environment, and as in conditions such as autism, hypertension, and obesity, ADHD symptoms are distributed along a continuum. By one estimate, 60 percent of the population has at least one symptom of ADHD (Arcos-Burgos and Acosta, 2007). Individuals with extreme traits and impairments tend to be relatively easy to diagnose, and they are likely to have had a childhood history of ADHD, said Sibley. But many of those who first present as adults have milder symptoms, which makes it challenging for clinicians to assess if these individuals have severe enough symptoms for an ADHD diagnosis, she said.

Clinicians may have different opinions regarding the degree of impairment needed to get an ADHD diagnosis, said Sibley. Individuals may report chronic self-esteem problems and feelings of inadequacy, which are considered mild impairments and difficult for clinicians to assess, she said. Clinicians can gain clarity on these questions if they follow best practices in the diagnosis of adult ADHD, said Sibley, but as the survey that Childress presented demonstrates, many clinicians do not follow best practices.

Ramsay emphasized the ripple effects that the disease has on adult roles and relationships with spouses, children, friends, and coworkers. "There are a whole host of effects that make coping with ADHD in adulthood very daunting," he said. Yet those affects may not always make a straightforward case for diagnosis and treatment. For example, "If your marriage is falling apart but your friends like you and you kept your job—or you're losing your job and everybody else likes you—is that enough impairment to warrant . . . a diagnosis under DSM?" he asked.

These uncertainties show why objective assessment is important, said Sara Weisenbach, associate professor of psychology in psychiatry at Harvard Medical School and chief of neuropsychology at McLean Hospital. Even if a person does not report significant impairment, a 20-minute continuous performance test may reveal observations, reaction time, or errors. Weisenbach noted that while some things can be difficult to assess by informal observation alone, at the same time, the subtle indications of ADHD can crop up during clinical interviews. Clinicians should be aware of subtleties, such as an individual's feeling like they have to work harder than their peers, as they work to obtain a more objective assessment.

One source of misdiagnosis, said Goodman, is "a presumption that treatment confirms diagnosis," which is incorrect (Zametkin and Ernst, 1999). A positive response to stimulant medication does not confirm the diagnosis of ADHD; it "just means that you altered [the patient's] brain chemistry, and [their] psychological experience is heightened mood, cognition, and energy." The converse is also true: failure to respond to a stimulant medication does not mean that the patient does not have ADHD. This is a problem, he said, because clinicians who do not make an accurate diagnosis with a comprehensive psychiatric evaluation may prescribe a stimulant to see if it works and continue to prescribe it when the patient returns saying they are functioning better.

Additional Clinical Features of Adult ADHD

There is a long-standing challenge in diagnosing ADHD, said Steve Lee, professor of psychology and director of clinical psychology training at the University of California, Los Angeles, in that many symptoms are not unique to ADHD but instead may be defining for anxiety, mood disturbance, or other disorders. Noting the "delicate balance" between the need to better define ADHD and the risk of adding so many other features that nearly everyone gets a diagnosis, he asked which clinical features of ADHD should be considered or studied further.

Executive function is "imperative," said Higgins, noting that many adult patients have problems with planning, prioritizing, procrastination, and organization. Emotional dysregulation is "the major drawback" that Tamara Rosier, founder of the ADHD Center of West Michigan and president of the ADHD Coaches Organization, sees in adults with ADHD, and it is common among Higgins's patients as well. People of different genders handle this differently, Rosier observed, contrasting two of her clients: a female surgeon who hides her ADHD from colleagues, and a male surgeon who expects that his staff will make accommodations for him.

Although the diagnostic criteria for adult ADHD address problems with concentration, the question itself needs refining, said Weisenbach. Activities such as video games that offer immediate gratification should be distinguished from activities such as studying that offer delayed gratification. Adults with ADHD may be easily bored when carrying out activities tasks that offer a delayed reward. This may be similar to delay aversion—an aversion to the interval of time between reinforcements—which is addressed by some of the interventions used to manage ADHD in children, said Lee. "There is something about the ADHD nervous system that is very different," said Weisenbach, citing work from the literature indicating that the vagal nerve and amygdala in people with ADHD are more "twitchy" (Robe et al., 2019).

The heterogeneity of ADHD symptoms is a big issue that further complicates diagnosis, said Sibley. Any of these additional clinical features may characterize one subset of ADHD but not another. Furthermore, when symptoms shared by people with lived experience of ADHD are compared to symptoms shared by people without ADHD, clinician often fail to differentiate among the two groups, she added. The symptoms may be worse in ADHD, "but unless there is a clear-cut differentiation, a clinician is going to be really struggling to figure out whether they have the disorder or not." In this respect, Sibley noted that "the DSM-5 symptoms have withstood the test of time," and while better symptoms are needed, "it's really a tough challenge to figure out what those symptoms are going to be."

Comorbidities, Trauma, and ADHD Diagnosis in Adults

The imperative against conferring an ADHD diagnosis if symptoms are "better explained by some other condition" conflicts with the reality that ADHD can co-occur with any of a multitude of other medical and clinical conditions, as well as the structural realities of time and resources needed to untangle the various threads of symptoms and causes, said Lee. How, he asked, can providers adjudicate the "not-better-explained-by-other-conditions" imperative while still accounting for the many other traits and comorbidities that can occur with ADHD? The problem of comorbidities is even greater for adults than children, noted Weisenbach, because untreated childhood and adolescent ADHD increases the later risk of depression, anxiety, and SUD.

Through her work with military populations, Brandi Walker, chief executive officer of Marie Pauline Consulting, LLC, indicated that she sees trauma as a significant comorbidity of ADHD. The trauma of the COVID-19 pandemic was a breaking point for many individuals with ADHD, said Taleed El-Sabawi, assistant professor of law at Florida International University. "There is a whole generation of women who were not diagnosed with ADHD," she said. "They are just being diagnosed now because COVID [destroyed] their coping skills."

Multigenerational ADHD exacerbates adversity, said Surman, affecting living conditions, accidents, interpersonal behavior, and parenting. Up to 17 percent of children with ADHD may have high prevalence of trauma or adverse experiences, a much higher rate than individuals without ADHD (Brown et al., 2017). "These different experiential or neurobiological problems seem to overlap very often," he said, and depending on their personal narrative, people may visit a therapist for trauma or a physician for ADHD, but given the prevalence of co-occurrence of these issues, it's important to have a "multimodal option of supporting people."

Treating Symptoms without an ADHD Diagnosis

Treating adult ADHD would be less stressful if it were possible to "step out of the diagnostic categories," said Sibley. Some practitioners will say, "If you have a symptom cluster, and I know a solution to that symptom cluster, then I don't need to think about the diagnosis—I could just treat [it]," she said. It becomes challenging when a diagnosis code is needed to justify the treatment. Practicing shared decision making, in which the patient prioritizes the symptoms that are causing them the most trouble, can also help focus practitioners on what to treat, she added. Without "these diagnostic boxes . . . we don't have to have these difficult decisions about which one is primary and which is secondary, we could just help people with what they need help with." Systemic factors "keep us using the boxes," she said, and that is part of the problem.

When a patient comes in and says, "I'm depressed and anxious," if ADHD is not included in the psychiatric comprehensive evaluation, the clinician will never see it, and the patient will be prescribed anti-depressants, countered Goodman, and the patient will still have cognitive complaints. To complicate things further, he added, cognitive dysfunction is also characteristic of many adult mood disorders. Providers must determine if the residual cognitive problems are coming from depression or ADHD after the depression has been treated. By only treating the presenting symptoms, "you've missed the opportunity to treat ADHD," Goodman argued. In a similar vein, Higgins noted that "poor attention is a symptom, not a diagnosis" and can happen for a myriad of reasons, which makes screening to rule out other conditions an "imperative."

Providers Are Not Trained to Diagnose Adult ADHD

Few, if any, residency programs have any focus on adult ADHD, said Goodman. There is a lack of treatment for adult ADHD "because nobody has been formally trained," he continued. A participant in the audience noted that ADHD accounted for zero of the 220 questions on the recent psychiatry boards.

Angela Mahome, staff psychiatrist at the University of Chicago, agreed. "I did not learn about ADHD in my general residency psychiatry, but fortunately, becoming a child and adolescent psychiatrist helped," she said. Mahome consults for a school district in a small town where children with ADHD were given a methylphenidate drug, the generic Concerta, which was not lasting as long as expected, wearing off in four to six hours. Teachers told providers that the medication was not lasting through the school day, so the children were prescribed Ritalin in addition to the Concerta. This resulted in kids' getting kicked out of school, she said, because the stimulant exacerbated anxiety. "If the clinicians know how the medications work and they ask enough questions or they listen to the patients, a lot of times the treatment would get better. . . . More needs to be done for clinicians to understand ADHD," added Mahome.

Mark Olfson, professor of psychiatry, medicine, and law and professor of epidemiology at Columbia University, noted that adult ADHD is "still a relatively recently recognized phenomenon" compared to child ADHD, and adult primary care practitioners vary in their familiarity and confidence. Whereas "pediatricians view uncomplicated ADHD as their turf . . . that's less true in adult primary care," he said; nonetheless, "a lot of the treatment for adults with ADHD goes on in primary care."

Tiffany Farchione, the director of the Division of Psychiatry at FDA/CDER, said dispelling old myths takes time. Discussions around adult ADHD began about 20 years ago, she said, but myths persist, like those that say kids grow out of it or only boys have ADHD. "It's easier to educate the uninformed [provider] than the misinformed," said Goodman. In support of this, Solanto noted that it is hard to find professionals who are willing and able to take her patients when they age out of a pediatric ADHD program.

Lack of Provider Knowledge about Adult ADHD

Based on her experience treating college students from across the United States, Mahome has discovered many mistaken assumptions about ADHD among providers. "Many clinicians don't realize that dose is not based on age, weight, size, or severity of symptoms," she said. Providers do not know that overshooting the dose of stimulant medication can lead to worsening of symptoms and increased side effects. Some clinicians start patients on a middle dose of stimulant instead of starting at the lowest dose and increasing it if needed. Clinicians also do not understand how different stimulant formulations differ in their kinetics and interactions with other drugs and even some foods. Mahome provided the example of drinking orange juice interfering with the absorption of Adderall. "Even with nonstimulants, you have to be careful," she added, describing a patient who had been sent to the emergency room after their pediatrician instructed them to simply stop taking their guanfacine, a medication used to treat both high blood pressure and ADHD, which if stopped abruptly can cause rebound hypertension.

ADHD Misdiagnosis and Health Inequities

In the school environment, young Black and Brown boys with ADHD are frequently misdiagnosed with oppositional defiant and conduct disorders, said Higgins. If these boys are not appropriately diagnosed, or if they do not respond to medication, "then it is [interpreted as] a character flaw." Black boys as young as five or six years old with ADHD fail to perform to their aptitude, leading to depression and even suicide at very young ages, said Higgins. These boys are often characterized by ADHD, another learning disability, and high intelligence quotient (IQ). They are very intelligent but unable to demonstrate their abilities in the classroom, and they constantly get into trouble. Racially, said Goodman, "I think that there is diagnostic prejudice amongst clinicians. The Black child does not get diagnosed; they just say he's a [problem]. And the White kid gets diagnosed because . . . we know he could do better, so he must have ADHD."

The type of language used in ADHD assessments is also a problem, added Higgins. Much of the language in questionnaires and psychometric tests is based on "northeastern, upper middle-class, white, Ph.D. language. America does not all communicate that way," he said. At the clinical level, providers can miss the cues in patients' anecdotes about their lives if they are speaking at different levels. These differences in language levels may be responsible for many misdiagnoses, Higgins added.

STIGMA, DISBELIEF, AND INEQUITY SURROUNDING ADULT ADHD

"We underestimate the degree to which stigma still exists with the diagnosis of ADHD, whether that's childhood ADHD or adult ADHD," said Baker. Baker has worked in other fields with doubts about the condition and/or stigma surrounding it, including hypercholesterolemia, osteoporosis, and migraine. In these cases, the medical community put considerable effort into educating people about the consequences of going undiagnosed and untreated, and over many years, the stigma and disbelief faded, he said. Obesity is another disease that was not taken seriously until the impact was quantified, said Almut Winterstein, distinguished professor of pharmaceutical outcomes and policy and the director of the Center for Drug Evaluation and Safety at the University of Florida. In contrast, "there has been resistance to [removing] stigma in ADHD over time that I have not seen in any other . . . disease state," said Baker. "If [ADHD symptoms] were represented physically, I think we would have easier access to medication," said Rosier.

However, Baker cautioned against assuming that "the answer is simply more education and more communication." He suggested that the widespread persistence of disbelief in adult ADHD may reflect a "solution aversion" phenomenon (Ariely, 2023). "If you don't like the likely solution to a problem, you're less likely to believe that the problem really exists . . . [so] if you believe that a diagnosis of ADHD means you have to be prescribed a . . . stimulant, then perhaps you're less likely to believe that [ADHD] exists at all," he explained.

Gordon acknowledged that there are a lot of questions around the validity of late diagnoses. "Why wasn't I diagnosed until my thirties? Maybe nobody was paying attention to me. It was a failure of the system up to that point. . . . There were huge struggles [in my life] before that." Ramsay noted that skeptics will say that people are looking for a short-cut, but in reality "adults with ADHD are working twice as hard for half as much, staying late at the office, spending weekends trying to catch up, to the sacrifice of other modes of well-being." His patients' goals are "pretty humble," he said—to have good relationships and good physical and mental health—and "quite achievable," based on treatment outcome research.

Rosier talked about the shame borne by many of her clients. "They're smart enough to get through law school and then they hit the wall because they can't . . . do their billing," she said. "It becomes a character flaw. The level of shame these professionals are carrying, trying to be normal, is exhausting. . . . I think we can do better. . . . We can start giving people hope and proper treatment," she said.

"We are having this complicated public discussion about whether the diagnosis of ADHD is an identity or a medical category," said Sibley. "A lot of [clinicians] tell me it's easier to just put 'adjustment disorder' on it than to really dive into what's going on and what's causing it."

Jessica Gold, associate professor in the department of psychiatry at the University of Tennessee Health and Science Center and chief wellness officer of the University of Tennessee System, said that compared to adult patients, providers are better at believing kids and assume kids are being truthful about their symptoms. "I think we need to carry that with us into [our interactions with] adults and not assume that everyone is reading the DSM and asking for stimulants because they want stimulants," she said. For Joseph Schatz, director of the psychiatric mental health nurse practitioner track at the University of Pennsylvania School of Nursing, who is also an adult with ADHD, just picking up his medication at pharmacies where he does not know the pharmacist has been "a really uncomfortable" and stigmatizing experience, something that numerous workshop participants acknowledged as also experiencing. Stimulant misuse has made providers skeptical toward people who are disclosing genuine struggles in their lives, and "we have to be really careful that we're listening empathically and hearing their stories," said Andrea Chronis-Tuscano, professor of psychology and director of the SUCCEEDS: Students Understanding College Choices, Encouraging and Executing Decisions for Success program for students with ADHD at the University of Maryland, College Park.

Nonetheless, in some respects "we have really advanced," said Goodman, who was warned that he could lose his license for prescribing stimulants to adults in the 1990s. Although stigma remains a barrier to treatment for many with ADHD, human resources departments in most major corporations recognize ADHD, "and they recognize the requirements to make accommodations to occupational situations," he said. Furthermore, the current generation of college students is "remarkably much more accepting [of mental issues] than someone in my generation—I think there is a tidal change here," he added. Schatz concurred that "we are seeing an amazing shedding of some of that stigma [among] our Gen Z friends . . . but some of it is absolutely still present."

Stigma of ADHD Crosses Race and Ethnicity

The stigma of ADHD plays out differently depending on the racial or ethnic context. Black parents may resist a diagnosis of ADHD for their son, said Higgins, because "what goes along with that is getting in trouble in school, being picked on many times by the teacher, by the school, and the higher risk of juvenile services and even incarceration for the rest of your life. . . . I've never seen a White mom cry with a diagnosis of ADHD, but I have seen Black mothers start to cry."

Racial bias, language, and stigma combine to cause misdiagnosis, for example, when the parent says that the kid does not have trouble focusing "when he wants to do what he wants to do" and cannot have ADHD, combined with a clinician not astute enough to probe further, said Higgins. Then, if the teacher calls the kid a bad actor, he is likely to receive a diagnosis of oppositional defiant or conduct disorder. A child with ADHD may be having problems inside the home, may be dealing with poverty, or may be an immigrant who does not understand the language, said Higgins. Bias against an ADHD diagnosis is widespread, agreed Goodman. "Asian, Black, and Hispanic communities psychologize the experience of psychiatric symptoms" but do not always admit that there is a psychiatric illness.

Inequities, Biases, and Lack of Access to Care

Young girls with inattentive ADHD are often missed, said Higgins, since ADHD does not often manifest as behavioral disruptions in girls. "There's a gender bias in the diagnosis of ADHD in females versus males," agreed Goodman, noting a body of literature that speaks to gender bias in the medical evaluation of women and that "girls with ADHD end up more likely to be on antidepressants than boys with ADHD."

Older adults face inequitable treatment due to diagnostic uncertainty and prescription hesitancy, said Goodman, while residents of rural communities are underserved due to a scarcity of trained clinicians and the difficulties of traveling to obtain care. "There are tons of disparities," said Mahome, and not just for minorities, as many assume that kids misbehave because of their background or socioeconomic status. For people with high IQs, she said, clinicians may assume that "if you did well in school, you cannot have ADHD." Mahome was diagnosed during her residency program, and she also noted disparities for women. Schatz treats patients on long-term disability and unemployed people "who are told they don't need their treatment because they're not working." He also noted the difficulties of getting treatment for patients with a history of or current SUD.

Kevin Antshel, professor of psychology and associate department chair at Syracuse University, noted that "there is great discomfort in diagnosing and treating ADHD on college campuses" (Thomas et al., 2015). Although 90 percent of college health professionals surveyed supported the use of stimulants, most college students with ADHD go off-campus to receive their treatment (Aluri et al., 2023), which is particularly difficult for first-year students who "are scrambling to find community providers . . . and it leads to the undertreatment of ADHD," said Antshel.

Many of Rosier's clients are doctors, lawyers, and others with high IQs who did not receive good treatment from local clinicians. Her clients receive medication education coaching to help them communicate with their health care provider "so that they can survive." However, only a small fraction of adults with ADHD are lucky enough to get this treatment. "We are missing so many people who don't have access," she said.

Like everything else, the general insufficiency of care for adults with ADHD is worse for those who are economically disadvantaged, and that includes a disproportionate amount of people with ADHD, noted Gordon. "There are a lot of hoops to jump through . . . [just] to get on a waiting list" to get evaluated, he said. He knows adults with ADHD who waited two years for an appointment. "It costs a fortune to get the diagnosis on your own, it's probably not covered by insurance, and we earn less than everybody else," he added. Just finding providers who are experienced enough with ADHD is a big hurdle, added Ramsay. Sokolowska said that FDA is working to improve access to treatment by further investigating the role of telemedicine.

El-Sabawi offered her own experience of growing up with undiagnosed ADHD as an encapsulation of a generation of women that has struggled without diagnosis or treatment. "I'm part of that generation, and they just did not think we had ADHD. . . . We had to develop our own coping mechanisms. We were thought of as airheads." Multiple times, she said, "I could have been referred and was not . . . probably because I'm a woman of color, also probably because of the stigma and stereotypes that women with ADHD are just flighty or not as intelligent as others."

Throughout college and law school, El-Sabawi missed several important milestones, but none of her professors suggested she seek help. After her brother was diagnosed with ADHD, she sought treatment and was found to have "really bad ADHD." She noted she was about 30 years old when she was diagnosed. "Imagine how much easier life would have been" had she been treated earlier, she mused.

ASSESSING ADULT ADHD: PRECISION VS. PRAGMATISM

Panelists explored the tension between the desire for precise psychometric measurements and the short time available to teachers and medical professionals for assessing ADHD in students and patients. "The amount you have to [bill] to keep the lights on and to make sure that everybody is paid [means that] everything in medicine is getting faster. . . . I know some clinicians who schedule patients every 10" minutes, noted Higgins. If providers are going to be asked to fill out a questionnaire in that time, the chance of it being done correctly is low, he said. Lee noted that "psychometrically speaking, measurement improves when we overmeasure . . . [but] that is going to be inversely correlated with the probability of clinical use." How, he asked, could the field negotiate the desire for precision and rigor of measurement against the time-strapped reality of primary care physicians and teachers?

The field could take advantage of modern psychometric theory by using computerized adaptive testing in scoring for ADHD, suggested Weisenbach. In this type of test, an early question would differentiate moderately positive from negative cases, and the next question would be selected based on the answer to its predecessor. This enables a much shorter test that would decrease the time it takes to identify positive cases, said Weisenbach. Development of these tools would be a good target for funding, she added.

Although psychometric measurements are relevant for identifying people who need a closer look, "a psychometrically sound instrument . . . is not the same as a good diagnostic tool," said Sibley. It is not enough to know the number of symptoms endorsed by the respondent. Self-reported symptoms are strengthened by collateral reports, even more than by performance on a cognitive task, which "can have a lot of false negatives," she said. "We also need to know about impairment, differential diagnosis, when the symptoms started, the chronicity of these symptoms, and the pervasiveness, and that is the part that takes so much time." Not all items should be weighted equivalently, said Lee. Conceding that few have the "time to use our best tools," Sibley nonetheless noted that "we have a big downside of them not taking the time."

"We need education to help people understand how to utilize these tools," said Surman, describing patients whose medical management was based solely on their score on a continuous performance task. Diagnosing and following patients using only objective testing measures is not sufficient, he said, because ADHD is defined behaviorally. Sunny Patel, senior advisor for children, youth, and families at SAMHSA, expressed concern that using objective measures to diagnose patients could create a bottleneck that filters out some affected individuals and delays treatment, based solely on their test score.

Solanto pushed back against dismissing standardized questionnaires outright. The Conner's Adult ADHD Rating Scale[1] and the Barkley Adult ADHD Rating Scale[2] were designed to describe symptoms as they are experienced in an adult context, she said. Scoring the longform versions of these tests produces an array of easily plotted symptoms, including "the DSM inattentive, hyperactive-impulsive, inattention-memory, [and] self-concept." Solanto finds these tests to be very useful and not too time-consuming, and her patients do not mind taking them. "I rely a lot on that to be able to validate the symptoms," she concluded.

Diagnostic Orphans

Because ADHD appears to exist at the extreme end of a continuum, as described by Sibley, it creates a problem of diagnostic orphans: individuals who do not meet the diagnostic threshold for ADHD but who are nonetheless impaired, said Lee. Considering that children and adolescents who fall just below the diagnostic threshold show persistence of symptoms and significant impairment later in life, participants discussed how adults in this category should be cared for.

The issue of diagnostic orphans reflects a need to re-envision what ADHD means and update the symptoms for adults, said Higgins. Many of his patients stop getting treatment when they finish high school because they do not see a need for it. "The ADHD doesn't bother them," he said, but then they start to struggle, and the current diagnostic criteria do a poor job of capturing their symptoms. Another hurdle, said Higgins, is the idea that "if it wasn't identified before age 12 then obviously you don't have ADHD." However, many individuals manage their ADHD symptoms as children, or the condition is not noticed. They may stay

---

[1] Available at https://www.wpspublish.com/caars-conners-adult-adhd-rating-scales (accessed March 5, 2024).

[2] Available at https://www.remedypsychiatry.com/wp-content/uploads/2020/10/BAARS-ADHD-questionnaire-PLEASE-COMPLETE-with-respect-to-symptoms-while-OFF-ADHD-medication.pdf (accessed April 26, 2024).

under the threshold until later in adulthood, when life catches up with them, he added.

Sibley concurred that "the diagnostic orphans of today may become the severe cases of tomorrow," noting that ADHD severity waxes and wanes over the lifespan (Sibley et al., 2022). There are risks to living with subthreshold ADHD, "and so we need to treat folks," she said. The problem that clinicians are having, she added, is that "in our system, you have to diagnose someone to treat them. It's forcing people to make choices about putting a diagnosis on paper in order to justify something."

On the flip side, in a world where people use social media to project ideal versions of their lives, "we are in this situation where people are being asked to do too much," and when they fail to meet unreasonable expectations, "they think it's because they have ADHD," said Higgins. This is a particular problem for women, who suffer feelings of inadequacy for not meeting lofty social, physical, career, and relationship standards, he said.

Impairment Due to ADHD

Worries about patients' faking it add to the stigma of mental health, said Farchione. If someone just reports a bunch of symptoms to the clinician that they can look up online, "of course you'll be worried about it," she said. "The difficulty is that in psychiatry, the symptoms of brain dysfunction occur in a psychological experience and . . . there is no objective measure," said Goodman. Even a knowledgeable clinician may be daunted when they see that an online search for "faking ADHD" gives more than 11 million results, he said. "How do I know the patient in front of me is not faking . . . and I'm going to prescribe a medication that's going to go . . . where I can't control?" These issues need to be addressed for clinicians, he said, for them to be comfortable moving forward in pursuing a diagnosis.

Symptoms can be faked, but impairment cannot, said Mahome. "Even people who are working on a PhD in astrophysics . . . can easily give me impairment, with car accidents and everything else, even though they were successful academically. . . . Most people don't know how to fake impairment to someone who is skilled at assessing for ADHD," she said. Patients who do not come into the office expecting an ADHD diagnosis are the ones whose lives you change, she added.

"It's almost a silent diagnosis in the adult population," said Walker, because ADHD is not obvious from the outside. But looking at patterns across a patient's lifestyle, you can see things falling apart even if the individual doesn't understand why, she added. Walker has to tell her patients that "executive function is all of your decision making . . . how you plan and organize, time management, the critical things that keep you employed or keep your relationships together." It is essential for clinicians to be educated about this, she said.

An Integrated Method for Diagnosing ADHD

ADHD cannot be diagnosed based on one test but instead requires integrating information from multiple sources, said Benjamin Cheyette, psychiatrist and director of ADHD programming at Mindful Health Solutions. His practice employs a battery of complementary tests, including two types of patient subjective surveys, one focused on childhood symptoms and the other on adult symptoms. He noted that each of these surveys has different strengths and weaknesses. The test results are integrated with information from the clinical interview and other aspects of the assessment. This integrative form of assessment is familiar to child psychiatrists, said Cheyette, but it is "all new" to adult psychiatrists. It is a process of getting people up to speed, he said, "but once you get that, it's pretty straightforward."

A Stepped Care Approach to Diagnosis of ADHD in Adults

To manage a huge increase in caseload at her former neuropsychological assessment clinic, Weisenbach developed a stepped care approach to screening and diagnosis of adult ADHD. For the first step, the referring clinician gives the patient a subjective self-assessment using a self-report scale of current symptoms (ASRS), obtains a childhood history to make sure that the onset of symptoms occurred in childhood, assesses for current functional impairment of symptoms, and if possible obtains a corroborative report. The ideal corroborative report would be someone who knew the adult well when they were a child, such as a parent or teacher, or even childhood report cards, said Weisenbach. If the screening measure and additional criteria are positive, the process goes to the second step.

For the second step, the patient completes an objective measure of ADHD symptoms, such as QbTest.[3] If this result is positive, the practitioner should consider and address any comorbid conditions, including medications that might have cognitive side effects, and readminister the objective assessment. If ADHD symptoms are still present, the process goes to the third and final step, which is referral to neuropsychology.

After implementing this stepped care approach, Weisenbach's clinic saw patients who were more complicated such as older adults and people

---

[3] See https://www.qbtech.com/adhd-tests/qbtest/ (accessed March 5, 2024).

with comorbid conditions. ADHD should be thought of as a public health disease and managed accordingly, said Weisenbach, by screening widely, outlining steps for managing positive cases, and giving access to specialty care, including neuropsychology, to those who need it.

4

Shared Decision-Making

Highlights of Key Points Made by Individual Speakers*

- Given the multiple possible treatment options and the need for individualized assessment of risks and benefits, shared decision making is a good paradigm for treatment of ADHD in adults. (Olfson)
- Social media contains both useful information and misinformation about ADHD that patients may turn to for medical advice. Providers can leverage these platforms by directing their patients toward reputable sources. (Gold, Walker)
- Medication provides a foothold, but it is not sufficient to treat ADHD on its own. Adults with ADHD also need to learn healthy coping strategies. (Barron, Chronis-Tuscano)
- Educating patients, teachers, and medical providers about ADHD in adults will require prioritizing and increasing access to structured, accessible, and trusted information resources. (Arria, Patel, Walker)
- To better track symptoms and monitor patient response to medication, measurement-based care should be used for ADHD in adults. (Cheyette)

*This list is the rapporteurs' summary of points made by the individual speakers identified, and the statements have not been endorsed or verified by the National Academies of Sciences,

Engineering, and Medicine. They are not intended to reflect a consensus among workshop participants.

Presentations and discussions about shared decision-making involved sharing perspectives and resources for prescribers, clinicians, and patients regarding treatment and management options for adult ADHD; practical approaches to working through barriers (e.g., stigma and misdiagnosis) to appropriately diagnose and treat adults with ADHD; and considering opportunities for shared decision making between patients and their providers.

ADOPTING MEASUREMENT-BASED CARE

Issues of cognition are treated differently than disorders such as hypertension, asthma, and obesity, said Weisenbach. Rosier agreed adding, "If your blood pressure is high when you go into your doctor's office, they are not going to say, 'Here, you need a hypertension medication.' They are going to say, 'Let's . . . monitor your blood pressure for a period of time, or come back for another visit so that we can reassess.' Why aren't we doing that . . . with ADHD . . . [or] other cognitive disorders?" She compared the care she receives for her asthma, which includes keeping track of symptoms and filling out a checklist at every doctor's visit, to that for her ADHD, which simply consists of her provider asking how she feels and giving her a prescription.

Providers need to monitor a patient's response to medication, said Cheyette. Current symptom-tracking measures for ADHD are inadequate, and while the ADHD Quality-of-Life Scale has been validated (Brod et al., 2006), it is long and impractical for clinicians to deliver to their patients before each visit, he said. Some clinicians use the ASRS, which is shorter, but it was validated as a diagnostic screening tool and not for tracking.

Cheyette developed the Hyperactivity, Impulsivity, Inattention Symptom Rating Scale (HII-5)[1], which consists of five questions, each scored between 0 and 3. Patients can complete the HII-5 in a minute or two, and they obtain a score from 0 to 15. This enables the provider to monitor a patient and track response to treatment across visits. "It's not meant to be exhaustive," said Cheyette, but it provides sufficient information "that you can quickly surmise how their ADHD is responding to your last medication change and make adjustments." The HII-5 scale

---

[1] Available at https://www.psychologytoday.com/us/blog/1-2-3-adhd/202306/tracking-symptom-severity-in-adhd (accessed April 26, 2024).

was modeled after similar scales used to routinely screen for depression, such as the Patient Health Questionnaire–9 (PHQ-9), and anxiety, such as the Generalized Anxiety Disorder 7-Item (GAD-7), he added. Cheyette presented tracking data from individual patients demonstrating the responsiveness of the HII-5 score to medical treatment for ADHD, as well as the overall correlation between changes in the scores on HII-5, PHQ-9, and GAD-7 (Figure 4-1). "There is a real need" for this sort of measurement-based care to track the progress of adult ADHD patients over time, said Olfson, noting that "a longitudinal perspective is very helpful in informing clinical decision making." The HII-5 is available for anyone to use, said Cheyette.

Reduction in PHQ-9 and GAD-7 in patients successfully treated for ADHD
(HII-5 reduction of 3 or more at follow-up; n = 30)

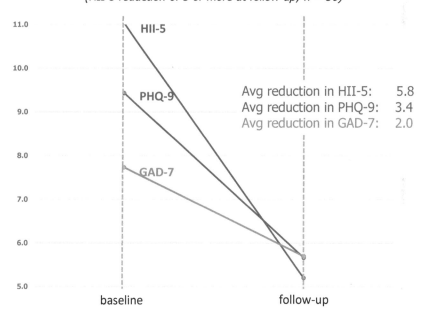

FIGURE 4-1 Tracking data from a patient undergoing ADHD treatment, comparing the HII-5 score to the PHQ-9 and GAD-7 scores.
NOTES: Graph shows data from one patent out of a group of 30. Avg = average; GAD-7 = Generalized Anxiety Disorder 7-item; HII-5 = Hyperactivity, Impulsivity, Inattention Symptom Rating Scale; PHQ-9 = Patient Health Questionnaire–9.
SOURCE: As presented by Benjamin Cheyette on December 13, 2023.

USING SHARED DECISION MAKING

Shared decision making is a model for the clinician–patient interaction in which both parties contribute information that is used in the clinical decision-making process, said Olfson. This includes decisions regarding whether to initiate pharmacotherapy, which medication to use, and what dose to use. Studies of depression have shown that shared decision making improves adherence with medication and improves outcomes (Bauer et al., 2014; Clever et al., 2006; Rossom et al., 2016), suggesting the same would be true in adult ADHD, he said.

Shared decision making can start with clinicians presenting technical information to the patient about the patient's condition, including the risks and benefits of available options, said Olfson. He noted that, given the information available online, "sometimes that discussion goes both ways. . . . People with ADHD often know more about . . . their condition [and] ADHD [in general] than their clinician." Patients inform clinicians about their goals and preferences regarding the consequences of treatment. All this information feeds into the decisions that are made, and "hopefully these decisions will reflect the priorities, goals, values, and preferences of the patient," he said. Obtaining the most robust efficacy may be paramount for some patients, while others may prioritize minimizing the risk of substance abuse. Ideally, Chronis-Tuscano added, providers "could engage in shared decision making regarding whether to begin treatment with stimulants, CBT, organizational skills, or non-stimulants. But limited mental health literacy may make this challenging in some cases."

Providing her perspective as an adult with ADHD, Kylie Barron described her experience with shared decision making. When she learned that she was pregnant, she stopped taking her ADHD medicine without talking to her doctor, out of concern that it might harm the baby. But after Barron left her car running in the garage and the gas stove on, her own safety became a serious concern. She felt "hopeless. . . . I've got to choose between me surviving and this unborn child surviving." Barron's doctor met with her to address these concerns. Over the course of a one-and-a-half-hour visit, the two worked together to review guidelines describing the risks of various ADHD medicines to the fetus. "I [was] able to make an informed decision about my own health after that appointment," she said. Adults with ADHD talk among themselves about self-empowerment and going to the doctor armed with questions, said Gordon.

It is critical for providers, especially general care practitioners, to take the time to talk with their patients and meet them where they are regarding treatment and diagnosis. "When we go to the doctor . . . there's not a lot of time left to talk about ADHD. I don't think I've ever told my doctor that I had four car accidents and ran somebody over," Gordon shared. That might have led to an earlier diagnosis, but it did not come up. If doctors were trained to ask and answer those questions, "there'd be a partnership formed that would lead to positive outcomes all around," he added. After all, Gordon noted, a person's ability to access the life-changing benefits of ADHD medication "all starts in that office with the diagnosis."

Cheyette agreed that poor training of practitioners stands in the way of shared decision making. Shared clinical decision making works best for disorders where there is more than one reasonable treatment option and a need to balance risks and benefits, said Olfson; furthermore, "there's a lot that we don't know [regarding] the lives of the individuals who present for care." For these reasons, he said, "the shared decision-making paradigm fit[s] well with the decisions that are often made in the medication management of adults with ADHD."

Adult ADHD and Healthy Coping Strategies

"There's a huge difference between treating someone with medication and actually managing a condition," said Barron. She compared medication for ADHD to drug treatment for diabetes. If you are on medication for diabetes, but then sit at home eating cake and candy, that's not managing your condition. With ADHD, she said, "medication isn't the final treatment. . . . You can use it as a foothold . . . but you can't expect medication to treat everything." Chronis-Tuscano agreed, and stressed that "it's really important to learn skills, like any other chronic condition. . . . It's not just about medication, but it's also about lifestyle, using skills, CBT organizational [skills], all of those [approaches]." Kofi Obeng, executive director of ADDA, added that "combining [medication] with things like therapy, group work, [and] behavioral modification . . . became force multipliers for me in terms of just having a better life."

After Barron moved and found a new provider, she was handed a list of rules, including limited rescheduling chances, no prescription refills if she was late to an appointment, and all her prescription refills must be requested within a week before she runs out. Barron asked herself, "Does she understand that I have ADHD?" Barron's provider told her that as long as she was taking her medication, "this should be pretty easy for [me] to adhere to." Taking her medication is the bare minimum. "It just gets me here," she said. "It doesn't help me find my keys or show up on time."

Medication can take the edge off, but it does not help a person manage life, finances, sustain healthy relationships, or deal with sexual promiscuity and substance use, said Walker. "We have people who take

ADHD medication and they're smoking marijuana every day," she said. "If they don't have healthy coping strategies, they will use whatever they've been using to get by." Providers need to make a concerted effort to help patients develop these strategies, she said, "and that is an ongoing conversation" that should encompass broader issues of lifestyle and may involve summoning help from others, like a spouse or coach.

"There's not a single answer here that's going to be right for everybody," said Cheyette, further accentuating the need for a broad-based conversation with the patient to determine how best to help that individual. Olfson concurred, noting that medications are tested on groups of people, but there is a lack of information about which medication and at which dose is going to be helpful for whom. "Even at the end of thoughtful and engaged conversations [with patients and providers], there is still an aspect of trial and error involved," he said, so "having some sort of therapeutic humility" is important.

"I think psychiatry sometimes focuses too much on medication" due to time constraints and insurance reimbursement, said Gold. She cautioned that medications can only do so much and that "there are other things people need to work on at the same time." Treatment is made even more difficult by comorbidities. "Sometimes medications never work," she said, referring to a patient who tried "virtually every stimulant . . . and nonstimulant" and never found one that did not worsen their anxiety. Having conversations about nonmedication management is important, she said. She is often able to help patients with referrals to occupational therapy, to learn skills for workplace management. "There are also a lot of apps for that," she added, and it does not take much time for her to show them to patients.

The U.S. Department of Defense has created "apps that give people access to just-in-time therapy," which could help supplement the care provided by medical professionals, said Walker. Wearable devices and other technology can also be leveraged for adult ADHD care. However, she added, "the bottom line still comes to resources, and being able to make sure that information gets out, and how practical it is for people."

ACCESSING RESOURCES

To successfully engage in shared decision making, patients and providers first need access to resources. Walker emphasized the need to standardize resources and help connect people with those resources early in life. "A lot of times that's not happening, so parents are struggling. And . . . without care, their children grow up to be adults with significant negative trajectories," said Walker. There need to be systems and processes for delivering these resources "to the people who are touching the people," she said: teachers, special education coordinators, and medical providers. Given the high incidence of comorbid conditions such as anxiety, depression, and sleep disorders, and citing her experience working at the intersection of trauma and ADHD, she said, "anybody treating those comorbid conditions should also be aware how the ADHD is undermining that."

Jonathan Rubin, chief medical officer and senior vice president of research and development at Supernus Pharmaceuticals, emphasized the need for patient education, particularly for adults with ADHD, "who may not completely understand the concept of ADHD as a neurodevelopmental disorder that persists throughout the day and evening . . . and potentially throughout their lifetime." Parents sometimes see ADHD as something that is only an issue during the school year, while adults view it as something that stops after they come home from work. "That framework needs to be reconceptualized, and patients need to be educated about the pervasiveness of ADHD," he said.

"Trusted messengers are really the key" for reaching individuals, said Patel, and the best messengers are often individuals with lived experience. Patel also emphasized the importance of instilling hope. "If you're looking for information and getting bombarded with disinformation, individuals who can provide trusted, accurate information that can also instill a feeling of hope are really important," he said. Following on Patel's suggestion, Solanto recommended a video made by the World Federation of ADHD that profiles individuals with ADHD (World Federation of ADHD, 2024), which she said would be educational for professionals as well as patients. She also cited the CHADD National Resource Center as a "good, important source of information" that takes "probably thousands of calls a year." SAMHSA publishes detailed manuals and guidance documents on ADHD, but these need to be turned into shorter documents that the public can use, said Patel.

The FDA could play a public education role by "translating into plain language what treatments are available that are FDA-approved for the management of adult ADHD" and making a concerted effort to educate the public about their importance and explain why medication is important, said Amelia M. Arria, professor in the Department of Behavioral and Community Health and director of the Center on Young Adult Health and Development at the University of Maryland School of Public Health.

LEVERAGING SOCIAL MEDIA TO EDUCATE PATIENTS

Gold primarily treats college students, and ADHD is one of the top three diagnoses that she sees. Many students watch TikTok videos about ADHD, she said. The TikTok algorithm is designed to offer more videos similar to whatever a person has watched already, so "if you think you have ADHD, you'll watch 10 more videos that tell you that you probably have ADHD." This becomes a self-fulfilling prophecy that leads Gold to hearing her patients say, "the internet told me I have ADHD." This might be correct, she noted. People who have never been diagnosed, including women and people of color, "will feel validated by what they are seeing." The provider's job is not to invalidate this experience, said Gold, but to "approach people with kindness [and] provide the information they're not getting" and offer to talk about it.

Gold shared the results of a cross-sectional study looking at content quality of ADHD videos on TikTok. The analysis of the 100 most popular TikTok videos on ADHD determined that 52 percent were misleading, 27 percent described personal experience, and 21 percent were useful (Yeung et al., 2022), said Gold. The study found that videos made by health care providers were the most useful and least misleading, which could make an argument "for [practitioners] to participate on social media," she added. Providers can leverage social media to educate patients and put out messaging "that reduces stigma and normalizes challenges with executive function," said Walker. It can "even [normalize] the concept of neurodiversity and [highlight] the strengths and creativity that come out of a neurodiverse mind." Some doctors do this very well, agreed Gold, who recommends these doctors' videos to her patients and encourages others to do so to update patients' algorithms.

5

Balancing Risks and Benefits of ADHD Treatment for Adults

Highlights of Key Points Made by Individual Speakers*

- Stimulants have one of the highest effect sizes (or magnitude of the difference) of all treatments, not just in psychiatry, but in all of medicine. (Goodman)
- Medical treatment for adults living with ADHD confers psychological, social, academic, and occupational benefits while reducing the risk of other negative health and social outcomes, even premature death. (Goodman, Gordon, Mahome)
- All existing medications for ADHD carry significant risks. Medical treatment requires a risk-benefit calculation, that may be different at the individual level than at the population level. (Sokolowska)
- The long-term effects of using prescription stimulants in adulthood are not well understood, and there is little information on the comparative safety and efficacy of ADHD medications. (Sokolowska, Surman)
- Insurance can interfere with ethical prescribing of drugs by requiring prior authorizations for extended-release stimulants and making patients try stimulants before they can receive nonstimulant drugs to treat their ADHD. (Childress, Rubin)
- Medication alone is not enough to treat ADHD. Cognitive behavioral interventions amplify the effects of medication. (Olfson, Solanto)

*This list is the rapporteurs' summary of points made by the individual speakers identified, and the statements have not been endorsed or verified by the National Academies of Sciences, Engineering, and Medicine. They are not intended to reflect a consensus among workshop participants.

Presentations and discussions on risks and benefits of ADHD treatment focused on what is known and unknown about ADHD medication use in adult populations; barriers (e.g., legal, regulatory, social, cultural) that patients face accessing equitable treatment; the public health implications for potential overprescribing of Schedule II stimulants; and exploring alternative treatment options (e.g., nonpharmacological interventions, retooling of existing medications, new drug development) that may reduce the risk of harm to patients while considering social and cultural factors.

CURRENT PHARMACOLOGIC AND NONPHARMACOLOGIC TREATMENTS

Pharmacologic Treatments

Based on data from 2020 (IQVIA, 2023), 61 percent of all ADHD prescriptions are for adults, said Goodman. Among these, 79 percent are for amphetamines, 13 percent for methylphenidate, and 8 percent for nonstimulants. Importantly, the prevalence of amphetamines is not because they work better in adults. Rather, he said, it is the result of marketing and education clinicians received after Adderall XR was approved as the first adult ADHD medication in 2000 (Heal et al., 2013). Goodman noted that most adult psychiatrists are not trained in child psychiatry or ADHD, and that nearly half of ADHD prescriptions are written by general practitioners or nurse practitioners (IQVIA, 2023), who know far less about the disorder than child psychiatrists or pediatricians. "You move into adulthood, and it is . . . the wild, wild west of psychiatry," he said.

There are currently more than 30 preparations for stimulant medication on the market, which is "mind-boggling," said Goodman. These comprise 7 stimulant compounds that can be grouped into 2 broad classes: 3 methylphenidates (racemic MPH, D-MPH, and Ser-dMPH) and 4 amphetamines (racemic amphetamine, mixed amphetamine salts, D-amphetamine, and Lis-D-Amphetamine). These 7 compounds are packaged into a variety of delivery systems, including beads (which may combine immediate-release and extended-release drugs at various ratios), osmotic release, microparticles (liquid, dissolvable tablet, or chewable), and transdermal patches. The delivery systems vary in terms of onset, duration, and side effects. Among the nonstimulant medications, 2 (atomoxetine and viloxazine ER) are approved for adults, and 2 (guanfacine ER and clonidine ER) are approved for children and adolescents but not adults, although they are frequently used off-label for adults, said Goodman (Iwanami et al., 2020). Nonstimulants may be used alone or in combination with stimulant medications, he added.

A positive response to stimulant medication does not confirm the diagnosis of ADHD, and failure to respond does not negate the diagnosis, said Goodman, noting that about 30 percent of patients do not respond well to the first stimulant and 15 percent do not respond well to the second, but this does not mean that they do not have ADHD (Rapoport et al., 1980; Zametkin and Ernst, 1999).

New Drugs in the Pipeline

Childress mentioned several promising new drugs for adults with ADHD. Centanafadine is a norepinephrine, dopamine, and serotonin reuptake inhibitor that has shown positive results in children, adolescents, and adults (Adler et al., 2022). Solriamfetol, which is being used to treat sleep disorders, had positive results in a double-blind placebo-controlled pilot study for treatment of adult ADHD (Surman et al., 2023). L-threonic acid magnesium salt may enhance synaptic plasticity in mice and has shown promising effects in a pilot study of adults with ADHD (Surman et al., 2021).

Nonpharmacologic Treatments

Some emerging companies are developing nonpharmacological treatments for people with ADHD, said Baker. The FDA recently approved an external trigeminal nerve stimulation device for children with ADHD (NeuroSigma, 2022). There is also an FDA-approved therapeutic video game (Akili Interactive Labs, 2024). Other modalities include ADHD coaching (Kubik, 2010) and CBT (Sprich et al., 2012). Each of these represents an alternative or complementary way to manage ADHD, said Baker.

This meeting underscores the need for nonmedical approaches to ADHD, said a workshop participant. Although the utility of coaching, CBT, and digital therapeutics has been suggested for decades, "you can't get the same level of treatment in the community . . . because it's not regulated, it's not delivered in the same manner," and it becomes a problem of access, he said.

Treating Adult ADHD with Medication

Before receiving an ADHD diagnosis, Goodman's patients blame their troubles on faults in their character, intelligence, and motivation. Diagnosis and treatment resurrect self-esteem, function, relationships, and sense of possibility, enabling them to "find a new direction in life, one that you never imagined you could undertake," he said. Goodman told the story of Maria, a 35-year-old Hispanic woman who came to see him for anxiety and depression. After a comprehensive psychiatric evaluation, Goodman diagnosed Maria with ADHD and treated her with long-acting stimulant medication and psychotherapy. Visiting Goodman three months later, Maria reported that she realized she was not mentally inept like her family had told her for 30 years. Obeng similarly shared that when he was diagnosed "it was a wonderful thing . . . being able to take medication opened up a whole new world." Treating ADHD "is unlike depression, where we return people back to their typical state. This is returning a person back to a state they never knew was possible," Goodman said.

Stimulants have one of the highest effect sizes (or magnitude of difference between groups) of all treatments, not just in psychiatry but in all of medicine, said Goodman. Individuals with ADHD experience significantly fewer physical injuries, car crashes, substance use disorders, and criminal acts, and improved academic and cognitive functioning, when they are taking MPH than when they are not taking it. "I'm Maria, and I am not alone," said Gordon. "There are thousands of us at ADDA who have a very, very similar story."

Medication Changes Patients' Lives

"ADHD is much worse than you think," said Gordon, an adult in his sixties with ADHD. "I spent half my life treated, medicated, and half untreated, unmedicated, undiagnosed. The second half was much better," he said. Before diagnosis and treatment in his mid-thirties, Gordon said, he totaled four cars and ran someone over. "It's expensive for me and for society to let us [with ADHD] operate heavy machinery unmedicated." He misused drugs and alcohol, was in trouble with the law, had career and relationship problems, and struggled with obesity and diabetes. "Think about how stressful my life is unmedicated," he said. "It's so much easier medicated."

Gordon described how the effects of medical treatment for ADHD ripple out. "The self-esteem coming back, the ability . . . to apply yourself to learning the different skills that you need to manage your ADHD, to diet, to get to the gym, to sleep better, to follow up with a specialist if you need to, all start with that initial diagnosis and the medication and treatment." Goodman agreed, noting that properly medicated patients have improved symptoms and day-to-day functioning, leading to increases in self-esteem and confidence. "It's an upward spiral," he said, that he sees in many of his patients.

Although Gordon's doctor worries about the potential cardiovascular effects of stimulants, Gordon is more concerned about losing access to his ADHD medication. Cardiovascular issues "can be managed medically. . . . I take a whole row of pills already for all the stuff that I have. [Adding] one more for cardiovascular issues scares me a lot less than going unmedicated with ADHD." He added that coaching and behavioral therapy are also necessary and that it is "not all about the medication." Nonetheless, weighing the risks and benefits of treating ADHD, he said, "I really want [the audience] to understand how heavy the side of not treating ADHD is. It's a huge risk."

"Treating ADHD definitely can save lives," said Mahome, noting the higher risk of suicide in individuals with ADHD. Describing her own experience during the stimulant shortage, which included rapid weight gain and resigning from her job, she said that when she is off her medication, she is "not the same person that I am when I'm on it."

The Two Sides of an ADHD Diagnosis and Treatment

Despite the benefits of treatment, there are arguments both for and against receiving an ADHD diagnosis and treatment, noted Goodman. Appropriate treatment for ADHD can be transformational, conferring psychological, social, academic, and occupational benefits while reducing a person's risk of negative outcomes such as SUD, tobacco use, car accidents, criminal behavior, unwanted pregnancy, financial debt, multiple jobs, and premature death, along with the societal costs they entail. But diagnosis can also have downsides, he noted, sometimes by making a person ineligible for insurance and for certain occupations. Treatment with ADHD drugs can result in testing positive on a drug screen, and the drugs themselves have a range of possible effects and side effects, including psychosis and cardiovascular changes. Use of prescription stimulants also carries the risk of misuse, abuse, or diversion. Additionally, if the diagnosis is incorrect, it may lead the patient to construct a false psychological narrative, he added.

Another potential downside to treatment for ADHD, noted by Higgins, is that some adults like their ADHD symptoms. Adults with ADHD can experience quicker processing and greater passion and drive, he said, and these traits can be advantageous under certain circumstances. Some patients feel that medicating their ADHD robs them of desirable personality traits. "We don't pay enough attention to that," he said; we might think, "It's a disease, illness, so therefore we must treat it." Higgins recommended that clinicians be more flexible with both the diagnosis and options for treatment, which "can go a long way towards engaging more people."

The cardiovascular changes caused by stimulant medications and atomoxetine are statistically significant but clinically small, said Goodman, and the small changes in blood pressure and pulse rate can be medically managed if the patient has hypertension (Cortese and Fava, 2024; Hennissen et al., 2017). Nonetheless, 5 to 15 percent of patients experience larger cardiovascular effects. "These are things that can be mediated by medical monitoring, balanced against the benefit" of treatment, he said.

Behavioral Therapy as a Part of Treatment

One of the first principles for helping adults with ADHD is multimodal treatment that includes nonpharmacological interventions, such as teaching effective coping skills and self-care strategies, said Olfson. Behavioral interventions are typically given in combination with prescription medicine, which often remains "the cornerstone of treatment," he noted.

CBT is a powerful intervention that complements medical intervention for ADHD by helping the individual develop new habits, ways of thinking, and consequent behaviors, said Solanto (Liu et al., 2023). CBT aims to give people "effective coping skills [and] to identify and challenge their irrational beliefs around their health conditions," said Olfson. It can help prevent them from catastrophizing and challenge them to build more adaptive functioning, he added. Combining CBT with stimulants has been shown to improve outcomes for patients with ADHD compared to either treatment alone, as was first demonstrated in randomized controlled trials in 2010 and has since been validated by other research (Solanto et al., 2010). In a randomized controlled trial of adults with ADHD who took stimulants, those who also received CBT were twice as likely to experience a reduction in symptom severity as those who received simple relaxation therapy, and the gains in overall function and symptom reduction were maintained a year later, said Olfson (Safren et al., 2010). New behaviors developed through CBT will be maintained, continue to provide reinforcement, and become autonomous for the individual without requiring continued direct coaching and support, added Solanto. "Medications don't have this sort of persistence," said Olfson. "After they stop, the benefits stop."

While stimulants can enhance attention and impulse control, CBT provides skills and strategies to effectively deploy those functions, said

Solanto. To illustrate the importance of this focus, Solanto cited "pivotal" work showing that the estimated lifespan of young adults who were diagnosed with childhood ADHD is 8.4 years shorter than that of young adults who never had ADHD (Barkley and Fischer, 2019). "Thirty percent of the variance in this outcome was explained by the trait of behavioral inhibition," said Solanto, "associated with lack of conscientiousness with respect to self-care, sleep, exercise, and proper eating habits." These habits can influence other outcomes like substance abuse, obesity, type 2 diabetes, smoking, accidents, and even suicide.

Ramsay has been adapting CBT for treating adult ADHD. Medications, he said, are "broadband treatments" that target the core symptoms, which may lead to enough functional improvement to suffice. But since "ADHD is a performance problem," psychosocial and other nonmedical treatments can address the condition in context, personalizing the treatment to the patient, he added. Solanto has developed and validated a CBT intervention to address executive dysfunction in adults with ADHD that she is currently tailoring for college students. However, although the research shows that CBT can confer enduring benefits, many professionals remain unaware of this, and it can be hard to access therapists who are skilled at delivering this treatment, noted Solanto and Olfson. ADDA members are "huge advocates" of behavioral therapy, said Gordon, noting that until he became educated on how to manage his ADHD, he continued to struggle even after receiving medication. There is an unmet need for behavioral support in addition to drug treatment, he added.

Medication Adherence and Patient Safety and Outcomes

Adherence rates are very low for all ADHD medications, said Baker. In a multinational study on adherence, fewer than 50 percent of adults with ADHD remained on medication a year after they started (Bejerot et al., 2010), said a workshop participant. The two primary reasons patients gave for stopping their medication are that it did not work and that it had negative side effects. Baker questioned the significance of this finding, citing an unpublished drug adherence market research study commissioned by Merck & Co. around 2001 in another therapeutic category in which a third or more of people said they had discontinued the medication because of concerns regarding possible side effects, despite not having experienced them.

"The single most compelling message" to promote adherence, said Baker, is practitioners' reinforcing to patients that ADHD is a neurobiological disorder, is well established, and is quite common. But many patients get a different message. "If you have doubts that the condition is real, and . . . other people are telling you it's not real, it does make you second-guess," which can lead to some discontinuing medications despite experiencing symptoms, he said. Many patients tell Solanto that their psychiatrist said to "just take it when you feel like you need it." She said this is just one example of how many providers are not well-informed about the issue. "When do you not need to pay attention?"

Compared to stimulants, it takes longer for patients to feel the effects of nonstimulants, which many do not have the patience for, said Mahome. Nonstimulants also need to be taken every single day, she said, which itself can be a challenge for individuals with ADHD. Adherence is a problem for all patients, and ADHD's reduction of executive function makes it all the more challenging, agreed Patel. Schatz has been taking Dexedrine ER since he was a child, and he stays on it because he only needs to visit his provider every six months. "I've been tempted to look at some of the longer-duration medication [but] the idea of potentially being referred out to psychiatry . . . and then having to go to monthly appointments . . . is a barrier for me accessing full treatment," he said.

The words that a physician uses when first communicating the diagnosis to a patient can significantly reduce adherence, said Baker. For example, people are more likely to resist starting a drug if they are told they will have to keep taking it for the rest of their life. But if the physician indicates that the patient will be evaluated on a regular basis to see if the medication is still necessary, the patient may be more willing to accept the drug and stay on it, he said.

Participants with lived experience shared strategies for improving adherence. Joining together with others who have ADHD goes a long way toward encouraging people "to own their ADHD and stick with treatment," said Obeng. ADDA has multiple support groups where individuals can find supportive communities they can relate to, where "you don't have to explain your trials and tribulations, people understand automatically . . . being able to find that community and that . . . brings so much empowerment," said Obeng. ADDA membership more than doubled since the stimulant shortage began, with people seeking resources and a supportive community, he added.

Systematic Barriers to Treatment

Childress said that 84 percent of clinicians who took her survey prescribe short-acting stimulants (Childress, 2023). She continued by saying that insurance "pushes [providers] that way," despite data showing that long-acting stimulants do not have the same potential for misuse. This is because insurance companies require prior authorization for nonstimulants, she said, which delays treatment. Additionally, prescribers are regularly audited for their notes, which can add hours of extra paperwork. Roughly half the clinicians in Childress's survey said that insurance pushed them to prescribe generic short-acting stimulants and refused to cover nonstimulants. Unlike pediatricians, many of whom have switched to using extended-release stimulants, adult prescribers predominantly use immediate-release stimulants. Rubin said these may not be appropriate in all cases, particularly in light of Childress's finding that most adults on stimulant medicine for ADHD were not completely satisfied with their treatment.

Patients' insurance and the medications it covers often determine what the prescriber will give, said Mahome. This is because many do not have time to do prior authorizations. For "no other condition . . . not schizophrenia, not bipolar, do I need to validate the diagnosis and go through a set of 15 questions. It's more restrictive, and that is stigma," said Schatz.

It is unethical to require patients step through a product that is less efficacious or more harmful than the intended product, said Rubin, but this is what happens when managed care dictates treatment decisions to clinicians and "gets in the way of the patient–physician relationship to . . . determine what is in the patient's best interest." Rubin recounted a recent call from a young adult patient who was forced to switch from Supernus's nonstimulant drug, Qelbree, which he had been using successfully, to a stimulant, despite concerns about side effects. In certain circumstances, the insurer will not approve Qelbree until the patient first steps through other drugs that are not even approved for adult ADHD. "That doesn't make sense," he said.

Insurance can also determine what type of provider a patient sees, noted Robinson, citing a preliminary comparison of patients on employer-sponsored insurance with patients on Medicaid using 2021 data obtained from the Merative MarketScan database.[1] Robinson analyzed the types of providers seen by individuals who had seen only one outpatient provider type for ADHD in 2021. Among adults with employer-sponsored insurance, 50.4 percent saw a primary care physician, 12.4 percent saw a nurse practitioner, and 29.6 percent saw a psychiatrist, psychologist, or psychiatric nurse for ADHD, "providers who most likely have specialty training in mental health," she said. In contrast 42.5 percent of Medicaid patients saw a nurse practitioner for ADHD care, 20.9 percent saw a primary care physician, and only 16.9 percent saw a mental health specialist. Robinson noted significant state-level differences in the provider types seen by those with employer-sponsored insurance. Importantly, for both types of insurance, more than half of adult patients received some or all of their ADHD care by telehealth.

---

[1] Available at https://www.merative.com/documents/brief/marketscan-explainer-general (accessed April 30, 2024).

BALANCING RISKS AND BENEFITS OF
USING ADHD MEDICATIONS

All existing medications for ADHD, both stimulant and nonstimulant, carry significant risks, noted Sokolowska. "The central theme here is risk-benefit assessment," said Winterstein. Risk-benefit assessments may be different at the population level than at the individual level, and the individual risks associated with a drug could render it favorable for some individuals but not others. Balancing these individual risks with population risks can be difficult when making regulatory decisions, said Winterstein. Risk-benefit assessments need to consider lack of response to treatment, minor symptoms that could be managed with nondrug interventions, or a predisposition that increases the risk of a particularly bad adverse effect. Furthermore, the assessment of risk-benefit or personal preferences when considering alleviated symptoms compared to adverse effects is critical.

Overall, said Childress, medications for ADHD lead to improvement in a variety of symptoms in adults, including driving, injuries, depression, suicidality, criminality, and SUD (Chang et al., 2019). ADHD drugs worsen bipolar disorder because stimulants can make people manic, so the bipolar needs to be treated first, said Childress. However, psychosis and seizure disorders do not appear to worsen.

Winterstein spoke about the two major safety risks associated with stimulant use for ADHD: risk of developing SUD and cardiovascular risk. On the risk of SUD, she said, more research is needed to separate the effects of ADHD itself from the effects of stimulants, as well as the relative impact of variables like stimulant type, dosage, form, duration of use, and patient-specific factors. Winterstein and colleagues found that "concomitant long-term stimulant and prescription opioid use is quite common, and opioid use is more common among ADHD patients who use stimulants than those who don't," raising "important hypotheses" that need addressing (Wei et al., 2018). Still, she noted, "it remains difficult to identify those patients whose ADHD treatment might result in [SUD]."

Regarding the cardiovascular risk, stimulants affect heart rate and blood pressure as a result of both dopaminergic and adrenergic effects, said Winterstein. In the worst case, this could lead to ventricular arrythmia and sudden cardiac death. Winterstein and colleagues were able to rule out this risk in children (Winterstein et al., 2012). "There may still be subtle effects, but . . . this would result in a huge number needed to harm," she said.   However, a recent study that evaluated the effects of long-term stimulant use in both children and adults from a large Swedish population found a 50 to 70 percent increased risk of hypertension and arterial disease, though there was no association with arrythmias, heart failure, or cerebrovascular disease (Zhang et al., 2024). "This is not minor," said Winterstein, noting that "blood pressure targets keep being lowered, as measures that used to be considered normal are now linked to heart disease." She also noted that about 10 percent of adults taking stimulants had preexisting heart disease (Gerhard et al., 2010), "and we know very little about the risk of stimulant use in those populations." Unlike previous studies that failed to detect this cardiovascular risk, the Swedish study followed a very large, higher-risk population over multiple years, with a median of four years. Winterstein's study, which followed a million children for an average of two years, failed to detect any effect because the risk for cardiovascular disease in children is so low to begin with (Winterstein et al., 2012).

Providers need more data to make patient-centered treatment decisions, "that's very clear," said Winterstein, emphasizing the need to compare multiple options, including nondrug treatments and combinations. Given the risks associated with stimulant use, she said, "we need to think about tapering approaches" as well as alternatives for patients with cardiometabolic risk factors or patients who develop hypertension. Patients themselves need to decide "what their preference is, regarding an increased risk for stroke or myocardial infarction versus uncontrolled ADHD." Making these difficult treatment decisions will require "more subtle and really very specific comparative studies that allow patients, providers, and regulatory agencies to make informed decisions," she concluded.

"When we evaluate the risk-benefit ratio of treatment for ADHD, I'd say we've had an experiment this past year," said Greg Mattingly, president of APSARD and co-chair of U.S. Psych Congress, referring to the struggles of ADHD patients due to the stimulant shortage. At the U.S. Psych Congress (HMP Global, n.d.), he said, "it's the number one public mental health issue we hear about. Not depression, not schizophrenia, not anything else. It's not having access to appropriate ADHD care."

Long-Term Effects and Efficacy of ADHD Medications

The long-term impact of using prescription stimulants in adulthood is not well understood. Sokolowska noted that assessments of ADHD treatments are typically based on studies that last less than 12 weeks. The efficacy of Adderall, a mixed amphetamine salt, was not systematically evaluated for long-term use in clinical trials before its approval, and the efficacy of Adderall XR, an extended-release mixed amphetamine salt, was established separately for children, adolescents, and adults in studies lasting only three to four weeks (Cortese et al., 2018). Sokolowska emphasized the need for more long-term studies on both safety and effectiveness of the various treatment options, including their impacts on behavior, cardiovascular effects, and the risk of progression to nonmedical use or SUD. The FDA published new guidance for clinical trials of stimulant medications in 2019 (FDA, 2019), recommending randomized, double-blind, placebo-controlled trials and at least one fixed-dose trial, without dose optimization before randomization, to get a better readout of safety, she said.

Studies rarely involve head-to-head comparison of drugs that would enable providers and patients to make informed choices based on comparative effectiveness and safety of the treatments, said Surman. He also noted the importance of placebo controls and postmarket surveillance. Additional knowledge gaps exist regarding the impact of telemedicine and best approaches to improve access to treatment, added Sokolowska.

Medication Management of Adults with ADHD

Overprescription and Nonmedical Use of Prescription Stimulants

Although two nonstimulants have been approved by the FDA for use in adults with ADHD and additional nonstimulants approved for use in children are sometimes used in adults, "the overwhelming majority" of adults with ADHD who are treated with medication receive amphetamine-based or methylphenidate-based stimulants as first-line treatments (Soreff, 2022), said Olfson. These are Drug Enforcement Administration (DEA) Schedule II drugs with a high potential for abuse and a black box warning about prescribing them to individuals with a history of SUD, but they remain the first choice for treatment because "there's stronger evidence for more robust efficacy," he said. Olfson illustrated this with data from two randomized double-blind studies (Nasser et al., 2022; Spencer et al., 2005) that compared either MPH or the nonstimulant viloxazine to placebo (Figure 5-1). Over six weeks, the group receiving MPH showed greater symptom reduction than the group receiving viloxazine.

The prescription of stimulants to adults has increased over the past decade, particularly to individuals in the 31–40 age range, said Olfson (Figure 5-2). The number of prescriptions to people in this age range rose from fewer than 6 million in 2012 to nearly 16 million in 2021 (IQVIA, 2023). Olfson questions if this was because that age group had been undertreated "and we're playing catch-up," or if it was because of misuse.

A study from southern France (Pauly et al., 2018) found that adults ages 25–49 were prescribed "dramatically higher" doses of MPH than younger adults or adolescents, said Olfson. These older adults saw, on average, four different prescribers and four different pharmacists; 60 percent were also prescribed benzodiazepines; another 14 percent non-benzodiazepine anxiolytics; and 39 percent were filling opioid prescriptions. Thirty percent

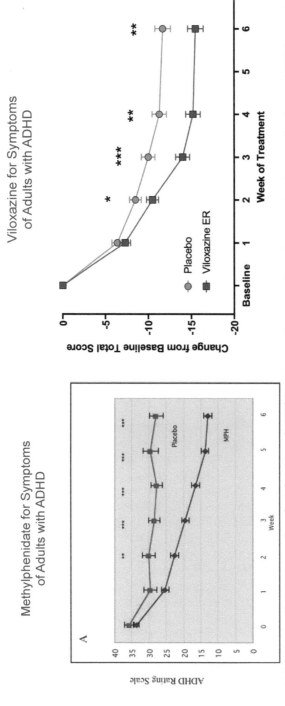

Methylphenidate for Symptoms of Adults with ADHD

Viloxazine for Symptoms of Adults with ADHD

FIGURE 5-1 Comparison of methylphenidate (MPH)-based stimulants or viloxazine nonstimulant to placebo on ADHD score in adults from two randomized double-blind studies.

NOTE: * indicate significant levels. On the left, * = p< 0.01; ** = p< 0.001; *** = p< 0.0001. On the right, * = p< 0.05; ** = p< 0.01; *** = p< 0.001.

SOURCES: As presented by Mark Olfson on December 13, 2023; Spencer et al., 2005. Copyright with permission from Elsevier; Nasser et al., 2022, CC BY 4.0.

57

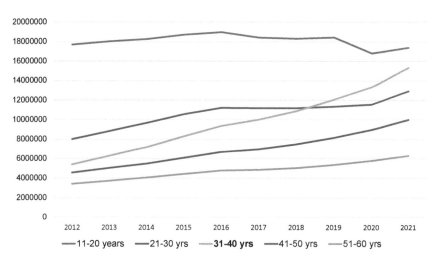

IQVIA analysis prepared for DEA, 2022

FIGURE 5-2 Number of stimulant prescriptions in the United States (2012–2021). SOURCES: As presented by Mark Olfson on December 13, 2023; figure created based on data provided in IQVIA, 2023.

of these individuals were filling prescriptions for methadone or buprenorphine, "suggesting that they have opioid use disorder," he said. A Danish study (Rasmussen et al., 2015) obtained similar results when it identified groups of patients who were being prescribed methylphenidate at doses "three times higher than what they call the defined daily dose. . . . I call it suspicious methylphenidate prescribing," said Olfson. The risk of being in this group was much higher for individuals in the 25–49 age bracket than for older or younger adults. Additional predictors for being in the high-dose-stimulant group included getting the prescription from a general practitioner or hospital doctor rather than a specialist, being prescribed benzodiazepines or opioids, and being prescribed medications for addictive disorders, such as buprenorphine. "Again, it's a concerning pattern that we see in opioid prescribing in this group," said Olfson.

Olfson emphasized the distinctions between abuse (using medication to get high), misuse (using medication in a way that is not prescribed), and nonindicated use (using it for purposes other than treatment of ADHD). One possible explanation for some of the increased volume of stimulant prescriptions, he said, is diversion: selling or giving away drugs outside legal channels.

One nonindicated use of concern, said Olfson, is when college students take stimulants as a study aid, or adults working in intellectually demanding professions take them as neuroenhancers. Studies of healthy volunteers offer some evidence that a single dose of methylphenidate can improve working memory, processing speed, verbal and learning memory, and (to a lesser degree) attention (Linssen et al., 2014). However, there is "very little evidence that these medications actually help with problem solving or reasoning . . . and no evidence that they help with visual learning and memory," suggesting that they might not offer the benefits students are after, he said. Nonetheless, he noted, "in some dimensions . . . these effects could be viewed and experienced as beneficial."

Increase in ADHD Prescriptions

The number of ADHD prescriptions in the United States increased from 50 million in 2012 to 80 million in 2022, according to DEA data presented by Sokolowska (IQVIA, 2023). In 2022, 90 percent of prescriptions were for stimulants and 10 percent for nonstimulants. Stimulant prescriptions increased over that decade by 58 percent, and nonstimulant prescriptions by 70 percent. This increase was driven by prescriptions to adults, predominantly females, in the 31–50 age range. The absence of adult ADHD clinical practice guidelines, coupled with the rise in both telemedicine and social media advertising of ADHD treatments during this decade, has raised concerns that some of this increase may reflect inappropriate prescribing, said Sokolowska. The COVID-19 pandemic may have also contributed to this increase, she noted.

Perhaps surprisingly, given the rise in U.S. stimulant prescriptions, studies have turned up no evidence of a corresponding increase in misuse, noted Sokolowska and Olfson (SAMHSA, 2023). According to the annual National Survey of Drug Use and Health conducted by SAMHSA, the proportion of people ages 18–25 in the general U.S. population who reported misusing stimulants actually decreased from 2015 to 2022. This level was lower for individuals aged 26 and up, with only 1 percent of that population reporting the misuse of stimulants. Nonetheless, in 2022, 4.3 million people in the United States aged 12 or older reported misusing prescription stimulants in the past year, and 1.3 million of those reported misusing prescription stimulants together with other stimulants, such as cocaine or methamphetamine. Looking more narrowly at SUDs, the national prevalence of prescription stimulant use disorder is about 1.5 percent of people ages 18–25 and 0.5 percent of those age 26 and up. "It's not a large number, but it's not trivial either," said Olfson, noting that in adults it's a fraction of the prevalence of prescription opioid use disorder.

"We still need to learn a lot more regarding the impact of nonmedical use of stimulants in adulthood," said Sokolowska, noting that plenty of data exist regarding the consequences of nonmedical use in adolescents but little in adults. A recent study (McCabe et al., 2022) found that the pattern of nonmedical stimulant use among individuals ages 18–50 follows one of six trajectories over time, with peaks occurring around age 18, 19/20, 25/26, 40, 45, and 50 (Figure 5-3). All misuse trajectories showed increased odds of developing SUD symptoms in middle adulthood. Based on their data, the study authors recommended screening for prescription stimulant misuse and SUD in adolescence and adulthood, said Sokolowska.

FDA is acting to curb stimulant overprescription and nonmedical use while at the same time trying to address the drug shortage, said Sokolowska, noting that label warnings have been updated to emphasize the serious risks related to drug misuse, abuse, addiction, and sharing. FDA and DEA are working in tandem to combat counterfeit prescription stimulants and to crack down on online pharmacies that sell Adderall illegally and pharmaceutical companies that do not identify the risks of taking stimulant medications in their advertisements, she said. FDA is also funding research to better understand the nonmedical use of prescription stimulants, she added.

Robinson presented information from a 2023 CDC Morbidity and Mortality Weekly Report on prescription stimulant fills using Merative MarketScan employer-sponsored insurance claims (Danielson et al., 2023), which was based on insurance claims data. The report showed a "sharp increase" in the percentage of adults receiving prescription stimulant medications during the first year of the COVID-19 pandemic (2020–2021). While there was an overall increase in the number of people receiving stimulant medication, from 3.8 percent to 4.1 percent of all individuals ages five to 64, the increase was particularly notable (i.e., more than a 10 percent increase) among adolescent and adult females as well as among adult males. It rose 17 percent and 12 percent, respectively, for women and men in the 25–29 age group. This kind of increase had not been seen prior to the pandemic, she added.

DIVERSION AND MISUSE OF ADHD MEDICATION

The treatment of adult ADHD creates several dialectics that need to be carefully thought through, said Patel. There is a tension between the need to prescribe stimulants where appropriate and the risk of diversion; between use of detailed, thorough screening tools that patients are unlikely

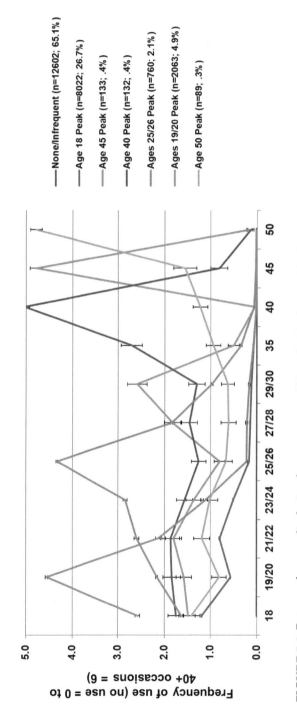

FIGURE 5-3 Pattern of nonmedical stimulant use among U.S. individuals ages 18–50.
SOURCES: As presented by Marta Sokolowska on December 12, 2023; McCabe et al., 2022, CC BY.

to complete in full or return and those that are more succinct but might not provide a full picture; between underdiagnosis and overdiagnosis, which vary based on population and setting; and between treating ADHD to prevent the emergence of comorbid SUD and the potential increase in SUD risk with treatment. Trends related to telehealth and online platforms for prescribing stimulants raise additional concerns. However, ADHD has serious adverse consequences, ranging from impaired academic performance to an increased risk of SUD, criminality, and death, as noted by Childress and many others. Therefore, Patel said, "individuals with adult ADHD need help, and these trends . . . should not preclude appropriate and adequate treatment."

Carlos Blanco, director of the Division of Epidemiology, Services, and Prevention Research at the National Institute on Drug Abuse, noted that this dilemma involves a risk-benefit calculation that requires balancing the individual's benefit of taking a stimulant against the community cost of its misuse or diversion. "How do we provide regulations and incentives so we achieve, if not optimal, at least second-best solutions?" he asked. This requires understanding how stimulants are actually misused and diverted.

Prescription Stimulant Misuse: Health Risks and Association with Later SUD

The risks associated with nonmedical use, also called misuse, of prescription stimulants vary with the route of administration, said Goodman (Faraone et al., 2024). The nasal route is associated with a higher risk of medical admission, oral with an increased risk of suicide attempts, and intravenous injection with a more than 20-fold increased risk of death; these data do not account for cofactors (such as comorbid psychological disorders) and therefore do not demonstrate causality, he noted.

The literature does not provide a clear link between early prescription stimulant use and later SUD, said Goodman (Chang et al., 2019). Animal studies demonstrated that exposure to stimulants during adolescence was associated with long-term risk of substance abuse (Kantak and Dwoskin, 2016), but more recent clinical studies found that ADHD medication neither raises nor lowers the risk of later SUD (Humphreys et al., 2013; Molina et al., 2013). Pharmacoepidemiologic studies drawn from a prescription database found that "ADHD medication was associated with a lower risk of substance-related events over three years" (Chang et al., 2014; Quinn et al., 2017), he said. Goodman suggested that the discrepancies might reflect differences in how these three very different types of studies were conducted.

Stimulant Misuse

Misuse of prescription stimulants is a serious concern. Among the general population, roughly 10 percent of individuals misuse prescription stimulants over the course of their lifetime, said Goodman, and this should be considered the background rate when studying misuse in patients with ADHD. Data consistently show that extended-release preparations of stimulants have a lower abuse liability than short-acting preparations, and nonstimulants have no potential for misuse (Findling, 2008). Nonetheless, Goodman advised against eliminating short-acting stimulants altogether, which would decrease the flexibility of clinicians and patients to manage ADHD symptoms.

"It's also important to know that many people who misuse stimulants do it infrequently," said Brooke Molina, professor of psychiatry, psychology, pediatrics, and clinical and translational science at the University of Pittsburgh. She noted that in the College Prescription Drug Study, 84 percent of the college students who reported misusing stimulants at some time in their life said they had used them zero to nine times in the past year (Kilmer et al., 2021; Phillips, 2018). Most students who misused stimulants were doing it not on a daily basis but during stressful times, such as during midterms and final exams, she said. Misuse is more common in schools that have more stimulant prescriptions, more white students, higher parent education, and more reported substance use. Misuse is also more common among males, white students, and students with ADHD symptoms, lower grades, substance use, or (among young adults) membership in fraternities or sororities; it peaks in the 18-to-25-year age range, added Molina.

Stimulant use among children with ADHD drops precipitously as they age, said Molina, citing her longitudinal study (Molina et al., 2023) that followed stimulant treatment and substance use in children from the Multimodal Treatment of ADHD study (MTA) for 16 years (a 14-month randomized clinical trial of treatment strategies for attention-deficit/hyperactivity disorder. The MTA Cooperative Group. Multimodal treatment study of children with ADHD, 1999). At the study's outset, the children had a mean age of 10.5 years, with 57 percent taking stimulants for ADHD. The percentage of children on stimulants dropped to 7.4 percent when the study group reached a mean age of 25 (Figure 5-4). This drop is commonly seen in longitudinal studies and suggests that children who are prescribed stimulants will not become addicted to them, said Molina.

As stimulant use among the MTA population declined over time, use of other substances like cigarettes, marijuana, and alcohol tended to rise. Molina found that children with ADHD had an elevated risk for harmful use of other substances, which is "a typical pattern," but this risk was not

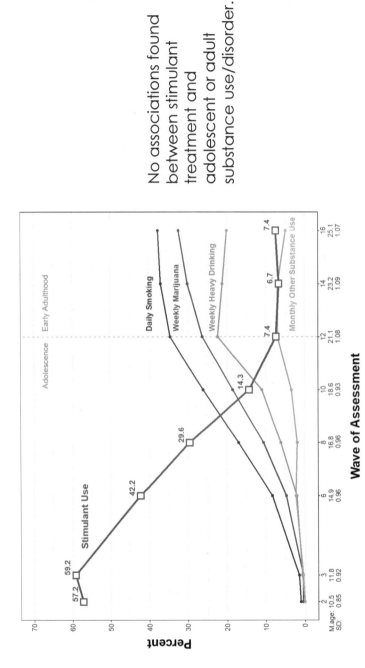

FIGURE 5-4 Association between stimulant treatment and substance use through adolescence into early adulthood.
NOTE: M.age = mean age; SD = standard deviation.
SOURCES: As presented by Brooke Molina on December 13, 2023; Molina et al., 2023. Reproduced with permission from JAMA Psychiatry. Copyright © American Medical Association. All rights reserved, including those for text and data mining, AI training, and similar technologies.

associated with stimulant use in childhood, "which was a great find," she said.

Higgins indicated that many of his patients who attend college report smoking marijuana on a regular basis, behavior patterns supported by the literature (Jean et al., 2022; Rooney et al., 2011). Students stop taking their ADHD medicine and turn to marijuana because they hear that it enhances dopamine. "But the fact is that you blow right past your dopamine levels to inattentiveness because you are dopamine depleted," he said. Higgins now asks patients whether they smoke marijuana, and how much, as part of his diagnosis.

Diversion and Misuse of Stimulants by Students

Misuse of stimulants is common among students, said Molina. In the 2018 College Prescription Drug Study (Faraone et al., 2020; Phillips, 2018), which surveyed 19,000 college students, 15.9 percent reported stimulant misuse at some point in the past, and 10 percent reported misuse in the last year. The Monitoring the Future Study (McCabe et al., 2023; Teter et al., 2020) sampled 230,000 secondary school students across the United States between 2005 and 2020 and found that 3.6 percent of 8th graders, 6.5 percent of 10th graders, and 7.2 percent of 12th graders reported misusing stimulants in the past year. This increase in misuse with age is "relevant . . . particularly with respect to prevention," said Molina. Nonprescribed use of stimulants varies widely across schools, ranging from 0 to more than 25 percent of students, "so one school is not the same as the next," she added.

The most common reason why individuals misuse stimulant medications is to improve academic performance, said Molina. Students take them to stay "awake longer, to pay attention, to have their arousal level increased, thinking that they're smarter," she said. However, research does not bear out this effect. In a study where adults with ADHD were asked to perform a complicated cognitive task with and without stimulants (Bowman et al., 2023), the level of effort increased but quality decreased when stimulants were used, said Molina, "so it's not a smart pill. . . . People often think that it does more than it really does."

In a longitudinal study of 1,253 college students, Amelia Arria and colleagues found that most nonmedical prescription stimulant use was associated with binge drinking and cannabis use, and these last two were strongly associated with academic disengagement (Arria et al., 2008). Students were using nonmedical prescription stimulants "as a shortcut or a compensatory mechanism" to address the academic fallout from drinking and smoking marijuana, said Arria.

College students constitute the highest-risk group for nonmedical use of stimulants, said Antshel. Citing nine separate surveys of college students (Advokat et al., 2008; Arria et al., 2008; Cassidy et al., 2015; DeSantis et al., 2010; Faraone et al., 2020; Novak et al., 2007; Rabiner et al., 2009; Verdi et al., 2016), Antshel said the primary motivation for misuse is that students view stimulants as an "academic steroid not as a drug, in contrast to "party drugs" like heroin or other opioids (DeSantis and Hane, 2010). Students also justify the nonmedical use of stimulants by saying they use them strategically and only during periods of high stress; or by minimizing the harm, comparing stimulants to coffee and energy drinks. The strategic nature of stimulant use in colleges was illustrated in a 2013 study, said Antshel, which found a jump in mixed amphetamine salts in campus wastewater in April and December, during exams (Burgard et al., 2013).

Citing another publication of Arria's that tracked stimulant misuse among college students over a two-year period (Arria et al., 2017), Antshel noted that students' grade point averages did not rise during the periods when they misused or fall when they stopped misusing, "suggest[ing] it's not the academic steroid that the average college student believes."

Diversion and Misuse of Stimulants by Adults

Not all diversion is done by college students, noted El-Sabawi. Diversion and misuse look different "for the adult population, the minoritized populations, disproportionately impacted populations." Indeed, long-standing work shows that there are moral economies of drug use, said Ryan McNeil, associate professor and director of harm reduction research at Yale School of Medicine, which are structured around sharing resources and supporting one another. Diversion of stimulants is often the result of sharing among friends, he said, "to support gaps in prescribing, lapses in medication . . . meeting gaps in broader systems . . . where we've let people down. . . . This doesn't happen in a vacuum." Furthermore, when diversion is considered against the background of a volatile drug supply that includes pressed pills, which may contain fentanyl or other adulterants that can amplify the risk of overdose, diversion can be protective, he added. Molina concurred, noting that most individuals who divert are not building up a supply with the intent of getting rich. "By and large [they] end up being approached, and it's hard to say no." Molina has worked with practitioners "to help patients anticipate those moments and have . . . a script" to explain why they cannot share their pills.

Terms like "diversion" and "misuse" suggest that drugs are not being used for medical reasons, said McNeil, but this may be a mistaken assumption about many of the adults who take stimulants without a prescription. He noted that "a lot of folks are using nonprescribed opioids for pain," and "extending that logic, it's reasonable to expect that similar dynamics are occurring here," with barriers to care or a lapse in care driving people to nonprescription use of stimulants.

Public health approaches to substance are "demand-side," said El-Sabawi. In contrast, the emphasis on diversion takes a "supply-side approach, which is typically focused on by law enforcement." Framing the problem as diversion, with enforcement as the solution, disproportionately impacts "people of color, people who are poor, people who are systematically targeted by carceral systems," said McNeil. "If we hope to avoid that, we need to reflect on what we're . . . constructing as the actual problem here." McNeil noted that engagement with the carceral system is an "incredible driver of harm at the individual level, at the community level, and society at large." Approaching the issue through an equity lens, he said, "we need to foreground that [harm] in the discussion so as to not perpetuate these systems that are so devastating to people and communities." Supporting this, Rubin offered that one option to address issues of misuse, diversion, and abuse of stimulants is to consider the prescription of nonstimulants as a first step when appropriate.

"People who are prescribed controlled substances will tell you that stashing is very important because pharmacies run out, you move, you can't find a doctor, you might be on a waitlist . . . or there's a restriction like you only have two days to fill your prescription," said El-Sabawi. Molina cautioned that doctors should not be "so tight on prescribing that [patients] don't have enough to carry [them] over from time to time," particularly in light of the difficulty that adults with ADHD have maintaining their prescriptions and getting to the doctor for refills on a regular basis. The goal of Molina's harm reduction approach (described in Chapter 7) is for providers to be aware if a patient has a lot of unused medication at home and to adjust the prescription if necessary, but not to prevent patients from having any buffer, she noted.

A public health approach should ask why people are using and stockpiling their drugs, said El-Sabawi. She noted that people of color may be less likely to see a psychiatrist, more likely to blame themselves for their disorder, and less likely to be diagnosed with ADHD, "and so we have over-representation . . . in the population using illicit stimulants who are people of color."

6

Potential Strategies and Implications for Drug Development

- Working within existing regulator frameworks, the market should be nudged toward nonstimulant options for adult ADHD. This can be done by focusing policies on efficacy, safety, and risks associated with misuse and diversion. (Lietzan)

*This list is the rapporteurs' summary of points made by the individual speakers identified, and the statements have not been endorsed or verified by the National Academies of Sciences, Engineering, and Medicine. They are not intended to reflect a consensus among workshop participants.

Presentations and discussions on strategies and implications for drug development focused on areas of unmet treatment needs for adults with ADHD that could potentially be addressed through new or improved therapeutics, and on challenges and opportunities for developing new or improved therapeutics for the treatment of ADHD, including options that may reduce the risk of diversion.

STIMULANT DRUGS FOR ADHD

The PFC of the brain supports higher executive cognitive processes that regulate goal-directed behavior, said Craig Berridge, Patricia Goldman-Rakic Professor of Psychology at the University of Wisconsin, Madison. ADHD is associated with a hypoactive PFC, and the core deficit associated with ADHD is dysregulated PFC-dependent cognition (Clark et al., 2022). "We've long known that psychostimulants are effective [for ADHD]. . . . [They] work rapidly, in less than an hour, to reverse PFC-dependent cognitive deficits," said Berridge. Developing treatments that work as well as MPH or amphetamine but carry a lower risk of abuse requires understanding how these drugs work in the brain, he said.

Psychostimulants act as catecholamine reuptake blockers, elevating extracellular levels of norepinephrine and dopamine throughout the brain when taken at high doses, said Berridge (Cools and Arnsten, 2022). When taken at clinically relevant doses, psychostimulants improve human cognition. Rats are a good model for looking at the biological mechanism of action, he said, and they show improvements in working memory and sustained attention, just like humans with ADHD, when given clinically relevant doses of methylphenidate (Berridge and Spencer, 2016). Higher doses lead to locomotor activation and impairment. Interestingly, when Berridge injected rats with MPH at clinically relevant pro-cognitive doses, norepinephrine and dopamine levels were more elevated in the PFC than in other areas of the brain (Berridge et al., 2006). Infusing MPH directly into the dorsal medial PFC, which is implicated in higher cognitive function, improved working memory (Spencer et al., 2012).

While MPH improves both sustained attention and working memory, the two functions have divergent dose-response curves, which reflects norepinephrine binding to two receptors ($\alpha1$ and $\alpha2$) with different kinetics, said Berridge (Figure 6-1) (Berridge and Spencer, 2016; Ramos and Arnsten, 2007). At the clinical dose of MPH that maximizes working memory (binding $\alpha2$), attention is only partially improved. But at the higher dose of MPH required to maximize attention (binding $\alpha1$), working memory becomes impaired (Spencer and Berridge, 2019). He suggested that this may explain earlier observations of target behaviors in children with ADHD on various doses of Ritalin, which found that performance on a learning task did not track with teacher ratings of classroom behavior (Sprague and Sleator, 1977). Similar effects have been seen in nonhuman primates (Rajala et al., 2012).

If cognitive processes have distinct dose sensitivities to MPH, this may have important consequences for patients, said Berridge. Although most of the clinical literature has focused on the therapeutic effects of dopamine in the striatum, he noted that all three classes of approved drugs (psychostimulants, selective norepinephrine reuptake inhibitor/atomoxetine, and $\alpha2_A$ agonist/guanfacine) target norepinephrine. MPH and atomoxetine enhance both dopamine and norepinephrine in the PFC, and considerable evidence points toward the PFC as a target for ADHD therapy, he said.

These observations have several implications for drug development, said Berridge. For one thing, they de-emphasize striatal dopamine. For another, they suggest that perhaps other molecules in the PFC could be targeted to improve cognition while avoiding the abuse potential of psychostimulants.

Pursuing this line of inquiry, Berridge noted that the PFC contains a very high density of neurons that produce corticotropin-releasing factor (CRF) in addition to CRF receptors (Hupalo et al., 2019). CRF has been studied for decades, but its cognitive action in the PFC was "virtually ignored," said Berridge. His lab found that CRF receptor antagonists elicit a significant improvement in working memory, comparable to MPH, while simultaneously improving sustained attention (Hupalo and Berridge, 2016; Hupalo et al., 2021). This suggests that "CRF antagonists may represent a useful approach for treating PFC-dependent cognitive dysfunction, including that associated with ADHD," said Berridge. He noted that CRF antagonists have been tested in humans for treatment of anxiety and depression (but not cognition), so they've already

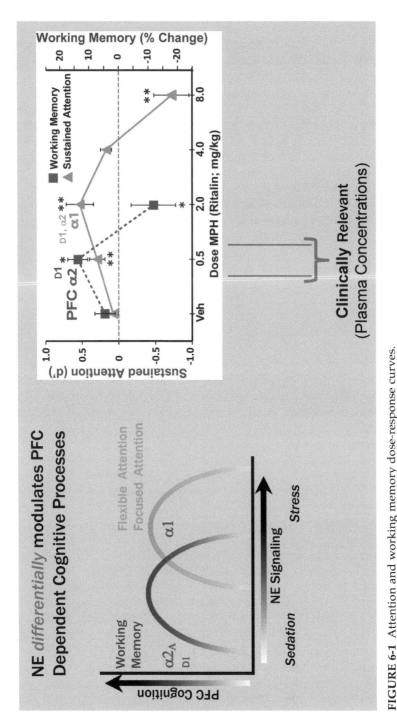

FIGURE 6-1 Attention and working memory dose-response curves.

NOTE: MPH = methylphenidate; NE = norepinephrine; PFC = prefrontal cortex.

SOURCES: As presented by Craig Berridge on December 13, 2023; adapted from Berridge and Spencer, 2016. Copyright with permission from Elsevier.

passed safety trials. "We should be thinking . . . a little more creatively . . . about what other molecules in the PFC could be targeted to reverse PFC-dependent cognitive deficit," he concluded.

NONSTIMULANT DRUGS FOR ADHD

A variety of nonstimulant drugs for ADHD, with a range of targets and mechanisms, are currently in use and in development. "We tend to bin all the nonstimulant medications together . . . but we need better terms to describe the medications," said Rubin. Citing Childress's data showing that only 29 percent of ADHD patients are completely satisfied with their medication, he said there is a need for alternative drugs to avoid the side effects of stimulants, to reduce the risk of abuse, and to address the current stimulant shortage.

Narrowing of attention has been considered the main desirable therapeutic effect of ADHD medication, "based on the old stimulant literature," said Amy Arnsten, Albert E. Kent professor of neuroscience and professor of psychology at the Yale University School of Medicine, but medicating ADHD offers other beneficial effects, including stabilization of attention and the ability to self-regulate attention, behavior, and emotion (Arnsten and Pliszka, 2011). These are functions of the PFC, and "many nonstimulants do very well in these realms," said Arnsten. However, many practitioners do not learn about the PFC nor know about nonstimulants. Arnsten cited evidence from rodent studies (Hains et al., 2015) that suggests the nonstimulant guanfacine "enhances the physical connections in PFC and protects them," raising the possibility that "we really might be fixing something . . . with these medications."

"When we hear that only 8 percent of adults are taking a nonstimulant, [it shows] how much progress we can make in that space," said Arnsten, who suggested making better use of existing drugs by "helping people to get through early side effects, starting low, slowly building up, and looking for improvements in prefrontal function, not just narrowing, so people know what to look for, what really might make a difference in their life, not just 'Can I get my taxes done if I stay up all night?'" Noting the importance of emotional regulation, Arnsten added that "the PFC has the connections . . . to control emotion thoughtfully," and this is likely to be helped more by nonstimulants than by stimulants, which risk activating the amygdala at too high a dose.

The Pipeline of Potential New Nonstimulant Drugs

There are new directions forward in developing drugs to strengthen the PFC without potential for abuse, said Arnsten. For example, partial dopamine D1 agonists, which have been shown to improve PFC function and are being tested in humans for Parkinson's disease and schizophrenia, may have utility in ADHD as well. Partial D1 agonists constantly stimulate the receptor, in contrast to the burst of dopamine that results from taking a stimulant and are therefore less likely to generate a reward signal that could lead to addiction, said Arnsten.

Arnsten's lab has uncovered additional potential drug targets, including the metabotropic glutamate receptor type 3 (mGluR3) and the nicotinic α7 receptor, both of which are important for PFC function in primates (Arnsten and Wang, 2020; Galvin et al., 2020). While the α4β2 nicotinic acetylcholine receptor agonist would have addictive potential, said Arnsten (the β2 subunit has been implicated in nicotine addiction), the α7 nicotinic receptor subunit has not been associated with abuse. Arnsten is also trying to tease apart subtypes of the noradrenergic α1 receptor to distinguish the one that helps with sustained attention from those that mediate stress-induced deficits in function. If she can identify the "good guy α1 receptor subtype," then it could in theory be targeted together with α2 (which enhances working memory) to improve therapeutic efficacy.

Arnsten noted that previous studies of the nicotinic α7 and dopamine D1 receptor, which did not show the desired effects, used high-affinity drugs that caused the receptors to internalize. But "these are receptors that endogenously need very gentle stimulation," she said. Arnsten's partial D1 agonists do this; "they actually mimic dopamine, a partial agonist by the same definition." Previous studies of mGluR3 caused confusion due to differences in the localization of receptor subtypes in rodents and primates, she added.

Rubin cited recent positive results on two triple reuptake inhibitors (targeting serotonin, norepinephrine, and dopamine): Phase 2 results on solriamfetol in adults with ADHD (Surman, 2021), and recent Phase 3 data on centanafadine for pediatric ADHD (Otsuka, 2022a, 2022b). Stevin Zorn, president and chief executive officer of MindImmune Therapeutics Inc., mentioned the possibility of targeting neuroinflammation, which he said is "a totally new way of thinking about ADHD."

Non-Stimulant Drugs Risks

Nonstimulants are not without risk, as several participants noted. Clonidine and guanfacine have "all the symptoms you would expect of a blood pressure medication," said Farchione. "You can have hypotension, you can pass out, [and] if you stop it suddenly you can have rebound hypertension." Some nonstimulants like atomoxetine can cause sexual dysfunction. Nonstimulants take longer than stimulants to start working and must be taken daily, noted Mahome. "Having the patience and hoping that you're not the person who ends up with sexual dysfunction or dry mouth or dizziness or any of these other things, if that works, then great. But if it doesn't, then it takes a long time" to see if patients develop those symptoms, said Farchione. Whereas it's easy to tell when a stimulant is "on," patients can have a more difficult time tracking whether their nonstimulant has kicked in, said Ramsay.

When atomoxetine came out, the starting dose on the package insert (40 mg) made patients nauseous, said Goodman. Clinicians learned to start at a lower dose and go up, but those who'd seen side effects induced at the package dose were reluctant to prescribe the drug anymore. While she acknowledged this problem, which has occurred with other drugs, Farchione replied, "if we don't have data from a lower dose, we can't put that onto the label." This is one of the reasons why the FDA is pushing for fixed-dose studies, which should make it easier to detect dose-related adverse events, she said.

BARRIERS TO NEW DRUG DEVELOPMENT

Bringing a new drug to market can take 10 to 15 years, said Rubin. It is a miracle that any drug gets approved, he said, given the bureaucracy that developers face with the FDA and other regulatory agencies, and the only way to justify the expense and time is if the pharmaceutical company views the product as a good investment. However, "managed care barriers can impede that," he said, to the point where few companies are working on ADHD because the generic stimulants are so inexpensive. "Even if you have a superior drug," he said, "the bottom line is that if . . . the generic costs a lot less, that's what's driving the decision."

Of course, it is much less expensive and less risky to develop variations of amphetamines and MPH than to do "a full-throated cradle-to-grave with a brand-new molecule," said Erika Lietzan, William H. Pittman professor of law and Timothy J. Heinsz professor of law at the University of Missouri School of Law. "That's going to create a little bit of hesitancy . . . to make that kind of investment," she said. One suggestion for overcoming this hurdle has been to conduct more early-stage drug studies, including Phase 1 trials, in academic settings. In addition, she said, the FDA should be encouraged to find ways to make Phase 2/3 clinical trials more efficient and less costly.

A barrier to new drug uptake is the absence of comparative head-to-head studies that would show the relative efficacy of new versus old drugs, said Lietzan. The approval standard at the FDA is safety and effectiveness, not comparative efficacy, she noted. Although policymakers and researchers are interested in comparative efficacy research, "I don't see the pharmaceutical industry pushing for that . . . but if we could get [comparative] data on these newer products, it could tell a very compelling story" and lead to reform, she suggested.

Managed care companies constitute a barrier "both for approved products and for future products," said Rubin. "A lot of pediatricians [are now] using extended-release stimulants, whereas adult prescribers are predominantly using immediate-release stimulants . . . which may not be appropriate in all cases," he said, but "clinicians are pushed [to prescribe immediate-release stimulants] by managed care formularies."

Cost vs. Treatment

When it comes to selecting a therapy for adult ADHD, "the primary focus is on cost, not effectiveness," noted Zorn, citing Childress's survey data. Arnsten wondered whether the cost of potential substance abuse is considered when calculating the cost of a cheap generic immediate-release stimulant medication. Rubin explained that three pharmacy benefits managers manage about three-quarters of all prescriptions in the United States (Mattingly et al., 2023). They provide this service to insurance companies but focus only on the cost of medication. "The insurance companies have to deal with both the medication cost as well as the cost of putting somebody in an addiction program, or paying for comorbidities, or paying for an emergency room visit because somebody got into a car accident," he said. In contrast, "the pharmacy benefits managers, who really control this whole process. They don't care about the overall cost of care, which society has to pay for."

Rubin cited a U.S. state that has "one of the worst stimulant abuse rates in the entire country," where practitioners were not allowed to prescribe his company's nonstimulant drug for their Medicaid patients with ADHD without stepping through a stimulant first. "That makes no sense," he said, because it limits access to nonstimulants "for the people in that state who have issues with stimulant abuse."

Developing New Drugs

MPH was approved in 1955 and Adderall in 1960, before any requirements for efficacy and clinical study documentation were implemented, said Farchione, and those requirements do add time for a drug to get to market. However, since "it's pretty obvious that stimulants work for ADHD," she said, companies have focused on "tweaking the PK [pharmacokinetic] profiles of existing drugs that we know to be highly effective." It is relatively easy to gain approval for a drug using the 505(b)(2) regulatory pathway (FDA, n.d.), said Farchione. "You can take an already approved drug and tweak it somehow with a new formulation, new dosage, new delivery method . . . change how long it lasts or turn it into a patch or something like that. And all you have to do is demonstrate that you can bridge" between the previous formulation's pharmacokinetic profile and the new drug's pharmacokinetic profile, she said. If the two profiles do not overlap completely, then clinical studies are required, but "those tend to be much smaller than studies that would be required for a brand-new drug," she added.

Reformulation of existing drugs led to the current proliferation of stimulant medications, said Farchione, noting that the clinical studies of these new formulations produced relatively little safety data compared to what is required for entirely new drugs (although a lot has been learned about safety over the many years that stimulants have been in use). Studies on these new formulations mimicked clinical practice, and "it was always kids" who were the study participants, she said. The dose was optimized for each child until the drug seemed to be working, then some participants had the drug removed (double-blinded) to see if it stopped working. "The only folks in that safety arm are the ones who already tolerated the drug," she said. To get better safety data, the FDA is now asking for studies of stimulant drugs to be double-blinded from the start with at least one fixed-dose study (FDA, 2019) "so we can get a true idea of the safety signal." Despite the difficulty of the approval process for some central nervous system stimulants, there are some brand-new drugs in development for ADHD that are not amphetamine or methylphenidate derivatives, said Farchione.

FILLING GAPS AND MEETING PATIENTS' NEEDS

Educating Practitioners to Prescribe for Adult ADHD Patients

The many different formulations of psychostimulants currently on the market have transformed the landscape of ADHD treatment for kids but not adults, noted Zorn. Physicians and nurse practitioners treating adults seem to lack the requisite education to offer patients the right stimulant formulations, he said, and they may not understand the advantages of extended-release stimulants over immediate-release drugs. Where pharmaceutical companies once conducted educational sessions for physicians, he said, there is now a void to be filled, and it needs to be filled in an unbiased way.

The NIH, FDA, or other nonbiased agency could develop a webinar that all practitioners would be required to take before prescribing medications for patients with ADHD, suggested Arnsten, "where you learn about the PFC and ADHD and the strengths and weaknesses" of existing treatments. This would apply to both physicians and nurse practitioners, she added.

Incentivizing Nonstimulants and Nonpharmaceuticals

Lietzan recommended working within existing regulatory frameworks to push drug developers and prescribers toward nonstimulant options for ADHD. The current regulatory framework for drug approval, labeling, and distribution focuses on safety and effectiveness and does not address risks related to misuse and diversion, she said. However, "there are some tools that the government can use to nudge the market" toward products with better risk profiles. Although stimulants and immediate-release opioid analgesics are "profoundly different," she suggested that the FDA's experience managing risks from the latter is relevant to the former. This included tools like prescriber education and guiding the market toward newer formulations. For opioids, "the boxed warning talks about the risk of abuse, misuse, and addiction and instructs prescribers to educate patients about them and to monitor the patients," said Lietzan. Putting similar box warnings on stimulants, as well as using funds that are currently available to the government for prescriber education, "can help nudge prescribers towards the non-stimulant option."

Payers are motivated by the cost differential between older, immediate-release generic drugs and newer products, noted Lietzan. It would therefore be helpful, she said, if governments and policymakers focused on therapeutic differences, differences in safety profiles, and differences in the risks associated with misuse and diversion. As far as legislation goes (for example, to address when payers can require prior authorization), "therapeutic benefits associated with newer products have to be profound and the focus of a great deal of education, including of policymakers," because affordability is foremost in their minds right now. Stimulants pose a problem of access in certain parts of the country because they are controlled substances, and that might be able to engage policy makers on the issue of reform, she added.

Baker offered further context on the current state of ADHD drug development and marketing. Two decades ago, he said, the leading industry players were large, profitable pharmaceutical companies whose annual sales of ADHD medications amounted to hundreds of millions of dollars, in some cases over a billion. These companies invested heavily in provider education and research. However, since their products went generic, they've all stopped investing in ADHD research and education, he said. The current ADHD industry consists of much smaller companies, most not even profitable, with very small budgets. Some are developing nonpharmaceutical therapies that insurers express a "befuddling" resistance to reimbursing, said Baker, despite the strong evidence base supporting them, and that makes it very difficult for these companies to turn a profit. Future efforts around ADHD education and research are unlikely to receive much financial support from these smaller companies, he said.

Developing Drugs Based on Patients' Needs

"Having a solid understanding of what the goal is, in terms of the functional action of a drug, is really important," said Berridge. He suggested starting with rodent models of ADHD but then moving to non-human primates, whose PFC functions more like that of humans. Based on work described at this workshop by Berridge and Arnsten, "there is strong reason to think that promoting PFC function without overfocusing it, [as occurs in] real-world situations, is a proven approach," he said.

Phase III clinical trials of drugs for ADHD enroll only patients without significant comorbidity, said Rubin, but such patients account for only 30 percent of all adults with ADHD and are "not clinically relevant to the patient who comes into the prescriber's office." Studying how these drugs work in patients with ADHD plus one or more comorbidities will be complicated, but it is a large unmet need for practitioners, he said, and should be explored.

Berridge noted the importance of reproducing results. His research on MPH was performed in coordination with other labs across the country. Reproducing experiments across multiple labs, using the same approaches and outcome measures, will generate more robust conclusions, he said, and this approach does not need to be terribly expensive.

Addressing the Shortage of Behavioral Therapy

The current medication shortage is not the only problem faced by individuals with ADHD, said Max Wiznitzer from CHADD. "The more chronic shortage is in the service delivery for behavioral interventions, which are much more difficult to institute and maintain," he said. "The medication can help you focus, but it's not going to teach you how to learn and . . . how to behave." As a consequence, he added, "we have a shortage of basically all the necessary interventions that are needed for both children and adults."

Solanto teaches CBT to trainees, but that's "a drop in the bucket," she said. To address the shortage of CBT therapists, graduate schools should train their students in this technique, she said. She suggested developing training and certification for CBT, as is currently done for dialectical behavior therapy.

A large-scale, randomized controlled study that demonstrates the efficacy of CBT could potentially change the landscape for treatment, said Solanto. She envisioned a study analogous to the MTA study that would compare ADHD medication and CBT both separately and together. There remain many questions about CBT, including whether some individuals respond preferentially to different treatments; how long the benefits of CBT last; and whether (and how often) "booster" sessions are needed, said Solanto.

There are evidence-based treatments, aside from medication, that teach skills, said Chronis-Tuscano, and that may be "an adjunct or even potentially a first-line treatment for individuals with adult ADHD." However, the workforce needs to be diversified to incorporate people who can teach these organizational and CBT skills, and providers need to be made aware and refer patients to them. Both Gold and Walker have referred adult ADHD patients to occupational therapy. "All those pillars—sleep, diet, nutrition, exercise, physical health, and mental readiness" were considered equally important for her clients in the military, said Walker.

7

Public Health Considerations and Harm Reduction Strategies

Highlights of Key Points Made by Individual Speakers*

- ADHD is a public health issue and can be managed by screening widely, outlining steps for its management, and providing specialty care where needed. (Robinson)
- Harmful use is not the same as abuse, and ADHD does not look the same in everyone. It's important to understand why stimulants are misused in a variety of populations. (El-Sabawi, Molina, Seliby Perkins)
- Adult ADHD needs an integrated treatment model, including collaborative care that partners providers across their professional silos. (Olfson, Schatz, Seliby Perkins)
- Racial and ethnic minorities are underrepresented in research, and little is known about ADHD in women, older adults, and gender minorities. Community-based participatory research should be leveraged to address these knowledge gaps. (El-Sabawi, Seliby Perkins, Sibley)
- The prescription stimulant shortage has been a source of chaos and harm, exacerbated by the "quagmire" of prior authorization, electronic prescribing, and rigid regulatory barriers. (El-Sabawi, Oliva, Weiss)
- Approaches to harm reduction could involve considering stimulant misuse and diversion against the backdrop of the illicit drug supply, which is volatile and dangerous; seeking

strategies to curb misuse by limiting the harms caused by engagement with the illicit supply; and understanding that untreated ADHD can itself be a cause of substance use disorder. (McNeil)

- Given the concerns about misuse and diversion of stimulant medications, perhaps newly diagnosed patients should be started on nonstimulants, along with cognitive behavioral therapy and organizational techniques. (Goodman, Gordon)
- The FDA and DEA should reconsider their strategies for curbing the misuse of stimulants, including rigid manufacturing quotas and restrictions on transferring electronic prescriptions. (Baker, Mahome)
- Training psychiatric residents, general practitioners, and nurse practitioners in ADHD treatment could include stimulant diversion prevention. (Arnsten, Cheyette, Goodman, Gold, Molina, Ramsay, Schatz, Solanto)

*This list is the rapporteurs' summary of points made by the individual speakers identified, and the statements have not been endorsed or verified by the National Academies of Sciences, Engineering, and Medicine. They are not intended to reflect a consensus among workshop participants.

Discussions on key themes from throughout the workshop focused on considering next step opportunities for improving the diagnosis and treatment of adults with ADHD through a public health lens, including harm reduction strategies to curb misuse of prescription stimulants. Blanco introduced this session by saying that what is needed is "a roadmap about where we want to go next."

A PUBLIC HEALTH APPROACH TO ADHD

The significantly shorter lifespan and health span of adults with ADHD (Barkley and Fischer, 2019), and the association of these statistics with unhealthy behaviors, indicates that ADHD is a public health issue in addition to a mental health issue, "and one that professionals in primary care need to be able to identify and address," said Solanto. Citing a 2021 Surgeon General's advisory that identified health misinformation as a public health threat (Office of the Surgeon General, 2021), Patel suggested that the amount of misinformation being circulated about adult ADHD itself constitutes a public health issue.

Indeed, the CDC began to focus on adult ADHD in the last few years using a public health framework, said Robinson. This framework describes a stepped process that begins by defining the problem on a population level, quantifying the prevalence of ADHD and other co-occurring conditions. Successive steps include identifying risk and protective factors, developing and testing prevention strategies, and working to ensure widespread adoption of these strategies. This is a cyclical model, said Robinson, in which each step feeds back on the previous step and informs the next, and a model that seeks to continuously improve access to information, support, and treatment.

The CDC has added three new items to its surveys to expand surveillance on adult ADHD, said Robinson. A survey using the NCHS Rapid Surveys System[1] should provide "very much needed new national prevalence estimates on adult ADHD," information from patients themselves on the role of telehealth in their diagnosis and treatment and estimates of the impact of the U.S. stimulant medication shortage on adults with ADHD. Results will be available in the spring of 2024, she said. Data from the recently completed DocStyles survey of providers should provide information on providers' comfort and knowledge on identifying and treating adult ADHD. Adult ADHD will also be included in the 2025 National Health Interview Survey, along with other questions on mental and physical health, to observe associations between ADHD and other conditions (NCHS, 2019). Additional potential content areas for questions include "diagnosis, type of provider who provided the diagnosis, severity and functional impairment, medication treatment, perceptions on effectiveness of treatment, telehealth, and . . . misuse and diversion," she added.

Adopting Ethical Principles for Prescribing Drugs

So that ADHD patients can receive medical treatment that is in their best interest and aligns with managed care pharmacy, it could be helpful for insurers to adopt ethical principles that have been developed by the Institute for Clinical Economic Review, said Rubin. For example, prior authorization should not require that a patient step through a product that is less safe or more harmful than the intended product; the first product in a step-through should have a reasonable chance of working. Managed care "should be asked to adopt these guidelines through accreditation, policy, or law, and bring that relationship back to the first party, between patient and physician," said Rubin.

Prescribing behaviors for ADHD have been influenced by the opioid crisis, said El-Sabawi. A public health approach to stimulant use should

---

[1] Available at https://www.cdc.gov/nchs/surveys.htm (accessed February 20, 2024).

seek "to understand how we can reduce the harms of stimulant use . . . with respect and dignity for all people who use drugs," centering their experience while "push[ing] back against the idea of drug seekers."

The Impacts of the Prescription Stimulant Shortage

The FDA announced a shortage of Adderall on October 12, 2022 (FDA, 2022). Based on preliminary data analyzed by the CDC (Danielson et al., 2023), the Adderall shortage may have impacted trends in prescription stimulant fills, said Robinson. She noted that children ages 5–14 receive mostly methylphenidate-based stimulants, and their prescription fills rose predictably during the third and fourth quarters of 2022, reflective of seasonal trends with usage lower in the summer months and higher during the months coinciding with the school year. In contrast, individuals ages 15–49 are more likely to receive prescriptions for Adderall and other amphetamine-based stimulants, and these fills fell during the same period.

The prescription stimulant shortage has collided with the quagmire of prior authorization to create a "mess of epic proportions," said Robin Weiss, past president of the Maryland Psychiatric Society. In Weiss's home state of Maryland, pharmacies are "entirely erratic and unpredictable" in their stock of stimulants, so that providers and patients often do not know which drugs will be available or in which dosage forms. Mandatory electronic prescribing prevents patients from moving their prescriptions from one pharmacy to another. As a result, the provider must submit multiple electronic prescriptions for each patient to find a pharmacy that stocks the drug. Mahome receives "tons of messages every day from students . . . asking [me] to send the prescription to a different pharmacy." Goodman relayed a story of a colleague of his who had to call 15 pharmacies to find medication for a single patient last week.

Rosier highlighted the irony of her clients' facing difficult or unnecessary tasks to obtain medication for their ADHD while they are off medication. The shortage has been "very real—it has impacted a lot of us greatly," said Mahome, who treats patients with ADHD and has ADHD herself. Mahome described her experience being off her medication for two and half months. "It's overwhelming having ADHD and not being treated," she said. She shared the difficult of dealing with a sudden switch from a 16-hour medication to one that she needs to take three times daily but usually remembers only once a day, "even with alarms." ADDA has done extra training "to help people deal with all the chaos that goes along with them not being able to receive treatment" and to educate people about nonstimulant options, "but it's been tough work," said Obeng.

"We understand the impact of the shortages," said Sokolowska, citing a joint FDA/DEA letter that emphasized how closely federal partners are working together with industry to address this issue (FDA and DEA, 2023). She noted that the FDA has approved new stimulant and non-stimulant medication for ADHD and granted authorization for the first diagnostic device.

Regulation and Access to Treatment

The regulatory barriers put in place to address the opioid crisis have created roadblocks that severely impact access to stimulant medication, said El-Sabawi, sharing remarks provided by Jennifer Oliva, professor, Indiana University Maurer School of Law, who was unable to attend. Because prescription drug monitoring programs are developed at the state level, said El-Sabawi, states "have different rules, different flags, and they are quite complex." Data on prescribing behavior are shared with law enforcement, and this engenders fear in physicians and a reluctance to prescribe any controlled substances. Some primary care practices have established hardline rules against prescribing stimulants and treating adults with ADHD, said El-Sabawi, noting that each physician's office has different rules, "and some of these go all the way up to the hospital-owned outpatient practices," where the hospital dictates the rules.

Given that filling stimulant prescriptions across state lines is complicated, students attending college outside their home states may have to establish themselves with a new provider to get refills on their existing prescriptions. At the same time, Gold said, "a lot of primary care providers [on college campuses] won't touch stimulants with a ten-foot pole." To ease this bottleneck while maintaining continuity of care, Gold advocated for universal licensing or telehealth prescriptions.

The rules imposed by state-level prescription drug monitoring programs also put pharmacists at risk, noted El-Sabawi. For example, in Florida, many state laws govern controlled substances. She said that pharmacies can lose their ability to order stimulant medications if they violate a state law, which could happen if they fill too many new stimulant prescriptions from one doctor. Further complicating matters, she added that "we don't truly understand the number of regulatory barriers because they differ by state," and interpretation of the regulations on the part of pharmacists can vary as well.

Distributors constitute another level of control, said El-Sabawi. After being sued over the opioid crisis, distributors developed proprietary software to monitor the supply of controlled substances. If this software flags a pharmacy, that pharmacy can be locked out from receiving a drug. This happened to the University of Miami pharmacy, which won a state contract to offer buprenorphine and as a result had a sudden increase in prescriptions, causing it to be flagged and locked out of receiving the drug. "There's no way around these new proprietary systems," said El-Sabawi.

In addition to state prescription drug monitoring programs, the DEA is "the elephant in the room," said El-Sabawi, with its own regulations, including a prohibition against transferring a prescription for a controlled substance from one pharmacy to another. Weiss noted that this rule was modified in August to allow patients to request a one-time prescription transfer, but none of the three pharmacies she contacted had heard of it.

Tension between Insurance Companies and Drug Enforcement

With insurance companies refusing to cover longer-acting stimulants and many nonstimulants, providers are being pushed to prescribe short-acting stimulants, but these are what are being criminalized, said Higgins. Furthermore, in the effort to shut down pill mills, law enforcement is targeting doctors. "It's a very real threat when you hear of a colleague where [the DEA comes] in . . . and [drags] you out to the parking lot," he said. This drives a fear of law enforcement that influences prescribing habits, and "we're not talking enough about that."

"The residents are scared to prescribe stimulant medication," said Mahome. "Those that want to learn how to prescribe stimulant medication might get an hour to meet with someone like me . . . but they're very discouraged from assessing for ADHD and treating it because of the potential risks."

While misuse and abuse of stimulant medications are a "pressing issue," Goodman warned against dealing with this by scaring physicians. "You, as a clinician, may read some popular literature that demeans ADHD in adults, that threatens your license because you are writing stimulant prescriptions." The uneducated clinician will respond by giving up writing prescriptions for stimulant medications. "And if I cannot write the prescription, I do not make the diagnosis," he said. These increased restrictions on medication "are being implemented in ways that discriminate as well," added El-Sabawi. Due to implicit bias, she noted, people of color are less likely to get opioids for pain and more likely to be identified as drug seekers.

"Before we start restricting access for patients who need stimulants, based on the fear of replicating the opioid crisis, it's incumbent on us— and by 'us' I mean researchers—to gather data on the actual prevalence of *dangerous* misuse of prescription stimulants. And I'm emphasizing the *dangerous* part," said Weiss. "I don't know if addiction is a huge problem with adults with ADHD," said Gordon; "mostly we forget to take it, which is really not a sign of addiction."

The Impact of Medication Access on Patients' Lives

Patrick Kelly provided his perspective as an adult with ADHD and a history of SUD. He had open-heart surgery as a young child for a congenital heart defect, was subsequently diagnosed with ADHD, and has taken stimulant medication for most of his life despite the cardiovascular risk, because the benefit was determined to outweigh the risk. Kelly described his childhood self as "hyperactive, impulsive, and lacking any form of self-awareness." He also had learning disabilities, and though he performed well on tests, his grades were low, and he was frequently sent to the principal's office. Kelly emphasized that the fallout of his ADHD was "not limited to childhood. I've lost jobs, missed opportunities, had failed relationships and various other things, and struggled with executive function as an adult." In college, Kelly discovered alcohol and often drank to excess "to numb the emotional pain that was caused by ADHD—the rejection, the disappointment, the constantly being told I had potential but finding it nowhere." Kelly used his stimulant medication as prescribed from age 22 to 23 but then stopped taking it at 24 and drank heavily for several years after that. Nonetheless, he said, "the stimulant medication helped stabilize me during those years, and it helped me get sober at age 26. . . . The two most important things I do on a daily basis are stay sober and manage my ADHD. The way I do that is through medication, support groups, therapy, extensive personal education, and building a life around systems, habits, and routines that address those two things."

Restricting access to stimulant medication threatens his survival, said Kelly: "When access to medication is restricted it puts my sobriety, and subsequently my life, at risk. When there's prior authorization, specific time windows, when it's classified as a Schedule II drug, or God forbid that I advocate for myself or state that I don't think this medication is working or that this dose is not effective, I am looked at as a drug-seeking addict instead of someone with a severe developmental disorder tenaciously and with good intentions trying to fit into a neurotypical world that is not designed for me."

The most important thing the FDA could do right now, from a public health perspective, is "to get people their medications," said El-Sabawi, noting that "more and more people are turning to pressed pills because they cannot access their ADHD medication, and they are going to the dark web." "Let's not do the opioid crisis again," she said, where "you close in on the supply of the prescribed medication, people go to the illicit market, and we get a spike in deaths."

Training and Clinical Education on Adult ADHD

Training Psychiatric Residents

For physicians to become better at treating ADHD in adults, "we need to get the educational professional programs to acknowledge that adult ADHD is a real disorder for which you need to train," said Goodman. The adult ADHD clinical practice guidelines currently in development seek not only to standardize care but "to standardize the validity of the diagnosis" and put pressure on accrediting agencies to get professional training programs to include adult ADHD "as a real focus for their curriculum," he said. Solanto agreed, "Even when we have such guidelines, we're going to need professionals who are trained and able to administer these treatments, and we . . . are far from having that sufficiently. It's so important that training in diagnosis and treatment of ADHD be included in residency programs, which it is not." This will require government agencies and organizations to commit "tens of millions of dollars of education," and a concerted effort by a body of experts to develop national coursework, said Goodman.

Gold noted that psychiatric residents are trained primarily in inpatient care, which consists of "a lot of psychosis, a lot of bipolar, a lot of severe depression," and very little ADHD. Given the paucity of even outpatient clinics focused on ADHD, this would likely require providing residents with specific opportunities to "see clinical cases with ADHD [and] make that a more specific focus for . . . residents with supervision."

Training General Practitioners and Nurse Practitioners

Arnsten highlighted the "great need" for general practitioners to receive education in adult ADHD. Given that many adults are treated by general practitioners and nurse practitioners, she said, "this information has to go back to medical school, nursing school," most of which "never even teach about prefrontal cortex," leaving clinicians ignorant of the mechanisms that underlie ADHD therapeutics. Many "practitioners and patients don't even know of nonstimulant possibilities," said Arnsten.

Noting that "a lot of primary care providers won't touch stimulants with a ten-foot pole," creating a bottleneck of college students waiting to see psychiatrists just to have their long-standing prescriptions filled, Gold advocated for shared responsibility: it "would be really helpful if some of those patients could be in primary care."

According to a recent study, the number of nurse practitioners in primary care is projected to exceed the number of physicians by a two-to-one ratio by 2030 (Pohl, 2023), said Schatz. That same study found that in the period from 2013 to 2019, the number of physician psychiatrists increased by 15 percent while the number of psychiatric nurse practitioners increased by 134 percent (Pohl, 2023). "This looks like a train that is not going to stop," said Schatz, and that makes it essential to "involve . . . the nursing voice and nursing perspective in everything . . . moving forward."

Training the Existing Workforce

Adult ADHD is a huge part of what adult outpatient practitioners are expected to do," said Cheyette. Therefore, patients "are often quite surprised" when their psychiatrist says, "I don't really do that, or I haven't been trained like that, or I don't know a lot about it." While this is "slowly changing," he said, "there's a backlog" of general psychiatrists and psychiatric mental health nurse practitioners with insufficient training in ADHD. To address this backlog in his practice, Cheyette developed a training program consisting of several required lectures that earn continuing medical education credit. Cheyette also designed resources for providers and supports them with monthly practice-wide case conferences. "That's all helpful, but more is needed," he said. Funding is needed for the national education of clinicians currently treating adult ADHD patients, agreed Goodman.

Given the current absence of adult ADHD from regular graduate or medical education, Ramsay emphasized the importance of training clinicians in the field. Training for adult ADHD remains "a niche specialty. You really have to . . . reach out to people," he noted. However, "once somebody [learns] the executive functioning model of ADHD and a couple of tricks they can use, the clinicians feel empowered," he said. "I've heard people say they change their practices [after] getting this information." For a practicing clinician, it would be more valuable to have algorithms than guidelines, said Blanco. Guidelines are necessary for specific cases, but few people will read a 40-to-50-page document, he said. Algorithms would be more useful "for people like me . . . to know what to do in most cases."

To illustrate how knowledge can impact clinical behavior, Goodman cited a comparison of electronic health records from adult ADHD patients in 2010 and 2020 that tracked adherence to 10 quality measures for diagnosing and treating ADHD in adults (Callen et al., 2023). In 2010 only 48 percent of records included 1 of these quality measures and 37 percent included 2 or more. By 2020, 90 percent recorded 1 quality measure and 75 percent recorded 2 or more. Treatment with a documented DSM-5 ADHD diagnosis increased from 52 percent to 97 percent over this period, and the number of patients seen within a month of their first prescription doubled. Other behaviors, such as checking vital signs before starting the prescription and discussing the warnings for medication, showed little or no improvement. "Some measures improve with education, some measures don't, which then goes to why we are doing the guidelines," he said. "While we're developing guidelines . . . it's important for us to get the information to [professional societies] that oversee primary care and behavioral health professionals," said LaTasha Seliby Perkins, assistant professor of medicine at Georgetown University School of Medicine, noting that the American Academy of Family Physicians is always looking for guidelines and tools to share with members.

Funding for Adult ADHD Education

When it comes to training health care providers to treat adults with ADHD, "who is the decision maker?" asked Zorn. He noted that Congress would need to give the FDA authority to extend the patent clock. But CHADD, ADDA, and other societies "with thousands of members with ADHD and associated caregivers" can influence regulatory opinion. Zorn suggested that "they and the rest of us step up and use these voices to call for this very high need for education."

Training needs to be funded by sources outside the pharmaceutical industry, said Goodman. "We need government agencies and organizations to [commit] tens of millions of dollars for education" and a nationwide curriculum developed by a body of experts, he said. In response to the opioid crisis, the FDA worked with medical schools to increase the amount of education regarding treatment of pain, said Sokolowska. She suggested employing a similar model to enhance practitioners' understanding of adult ADHD.

"A key message [from this workshop] has got to be education, education, education. How do we get it, who is going to do it, and who can take responsibility for that," said Zorn. "Give us money, we'll get education out there," replied Childress.

AN INTEGRATED TREATMENT MODEL FOR ADULT ADHD

Collaborative care models have worked well in adult depression care for training primary care providers and increasing their confidence, said Olfson. In these models, frontline primary care providers are paired with mental health specialists who they can consult when in need of advice. "Over time, there's a learning process that occurs," said Olfson, noting that pediatricians often say they have gained confidence from collaborations with specialists. Olfson cautioned that this is a "longer-term educational process."

The adult ADHD field needs to integrate diverse approaches to care, and there are models, like primary care behavioral health, that can help do this, said Schatz. Otherwise, the information is "great but . . . siloed," he said. "Non-pharm presents on non-pharm. . . . Psycho-pharm presents on psycho-pharm. . . . We're acknowledging the role for both, but I didn't hear about a model that integrates both consistently." One result of this disconnect may be seen in the data from Childress showing that "45 percent of clinicians were not able to identify the burden," he said. "That piece is scary to me, that we're potentially making this diagnosis without really understanding the patient's story." Schatz acknowledged health care providers' time limitations, but "we have also heard from multiple people . . . about the importance of taking that time." To build the capacity needed to address this problem, he said, will require "looking at alternative payment models [and] collaborative and integrative care. . . . We just need someone to build that integrated model that could be plugged into these frameworks."

Integrated primary care and collaborative care models work well for ADHD treatment, said Chronis-Tuscano. Working within these models helped Seliby Perkins develop skills in motivational interviewing, which she learned from training with behavioral health professionals. Thanks to the skills she developed, Seliby Perkins can educate her patients about their condition and engage in shared decision making in the span of a 20-minute visit. "If you sit down and look at someone eye-to-eye and actually listen, it takes less time than you think," she said. Furthermore, when a patient needs more than Seliby Perkins can provide, such as CBT, she has a team to refer them to. She emphasized the importance of "learning . . . from others, people on your team, and knowing when to send them to someone else."

Underserved and Underinsured Patients

It is easy to keep the focus on college students, said Seliby Perkins, stressing the need to "keep all of our patients in the conversation" and to understand the hurdles that need to be jumped for the underserved and underinsured. These are individuals who lack access to testing and cannot afford their stimulants even with a reduced cost card. "We're still fighting lots of stigmas for all of our racially underserved, marginalized, [and] gender-diverse patients," she said.

Seliby Perkins emphasized the need for all adults with ADHD to access treatment. ADHD is a treatable diagnosis, and appropriate treatment can enable a person to excel in their life, "whether it's a student or someone working at Safeway as a cashier. . . . They still have to be on top of [their lives]." If the child has trouble in school, the parent can volunteer that "maybe my child has this . . . because I have it. But if they don't know . . . then we're missing a lot of things in our society in general," she said.

Health systems need to figure out how to improve access and eliminate inequities while simultaneously ensuring quality of care that respects both patient preference and the evidence base, said Blanco. The insufficiency of provider training in adult ADHD care is particularly acute for members of underserved populations, who may not be able to access a provider with a high level of expertise (if they can access anyone), "and certainly not for an extended period of time," said Walker. For these reasons, it is crucial that all primary care practitioners be educated on medication options for ADHD, she said.

Higgins stressed the importance of educating the public about ADHD, including immigrants who may not speak English well. "We have almost no research on what ADHD looks like in individuals who identify as women, racial and ethnic minorities, middle-age and older adults, and sexual and gender minorities," said Sibley. This is contributing to "gaping health disparities." More research is needed into the role of hormones in the expression of ADHD symptoms and the effectiveness of medication, said Julia Schechter, a clinical psychologist at Duke, who noted that this is the main question received by Duke's Center for Girls and Women with ADHD.

"We need better normative data that is applicable to more than just the middle-class white population," said Weisenbach. This will require recruiting more minorities for research studies. The problem of minority representation in research data is not unique to ADHD, she added, and fixing it requires that scientists learn how to engage underserved communities. Engagement will improve when members of underrepresented communities become providers, but "it starts with an investment," said Sibley.

Seliby Perkins noted the value of shared decision making when addressing individuals from underserved populations. Seliby Perkins provides her patients with the same education as her medical students "because I feel they deserve the same information. . . . Here are the options . . . here's a handout, and we'll meet back and talk about it." Shared decision making lets her form a bridge "using cultural humility instead of competency because . . . I'm not going to be as competent as I think I am. . . . The patient helps you be more humble about the decision." It is important, she said, to take the information "and break it down into chewable bite sizes that everyone, no matter what their reading comprehension level is, can understand."

HARM REDUCTION STRATEGIES TO CURB MISUSE

Substance use must be considered against the backdrop of the volatility of the illicit drug supply, said McNeil, noting the "horrible unrelenting spike in overdose deaths driven by synthetic opioids." McNeil emphasized the need to limit harms caused by engagement with the illicit supply. This is particularly relevant in the context of the stimulant shortage, which may push people into buying pressed pills, "which seldom contain what . . . people think is in them," he added. Another element of harm reduction emerges from noting that college students often misuse stimulants to perform better in class or stay up late and get work done. "Why? What are the broader pressures that are driving this, and how can we intervene . . . to create environments that are conducive to learning, to living, to thriving, that aren't the hypercompetitive grind that people are on?" he asked, noting this broader context as "a point of intervention that we commonly overlook."

Patients in Jeopardy

Goodman cautioned regulators to carefully assess the evidence regarding the risks and benefits of drug treatment for ADHD when addressing issues of misuse and abuse, and not to "put the cart in front of the horse . . . while we restrict access and frighten clinicians from prescribing medications."

George Black, an attendee with lived experience, emphasized the wide-ranging benefits of stimulant medications for ADHD. He cited a recent study that found that diagnosis of adult ADHD correlated with an increased risk of dementia, but only in adults who did not receive stimulant medication (Levine et al., 2023), and another study that found that stimulant medication reduces suicidality in people with ADHD and bipolar disorder (Öhlund et al., 2020). He also noted a finding that the nonstimulant guanfacine reduced alcohol intake in rats (Fredriksson et al., 2015), and promising results from using guanfacine in combination with a methylphenidate stimulant (Michelini et al., 2023). Black himself nearly died in a car wreck due to unmedicated ADHD. "You don't want to throw out the baby with the bathwater," he said, cautioning against emphasizing the dangers of stimulants over their benefits. He noted that many of the worst adverse events caused by untreated ADHD, "suicide and car wrecks and all that . . . that's adults, generally . . . [and] there's not much discipline for underdiagnosis." Black sought assurance that the APSARD guidelines would counter many providers' reluctance to prescribe medications for ADHD when appropriate. El-Sabawi expressed a similar concern, noting that as a result of the opioid crackdown, patients with hysterectomies are "being prescribed Tylenol and that's the hospital policy. . . . We fear the same thing will happen with stimulants. . . . We have to be cautious about the narrative so we don't get the same policy outcomes."

Reconsidering Strategies for Curbing Misuse

Although the FDA does not control the supply of stimulants and therefore cannot directly address the shortage, it works closely with the DEA, which "has a big influence here," said Baker. One role of the DEA is to limit how much controlled substances are made and set "a quota for the total amount of amphetamine and methylphenidate that can be manufactured in the country." This is then allocated among the various manufacturers. The problem, Baker said, is that when one manufacturer has a problem meeting its quota, "other companies can't step in because their [annual manufacturing] quotas have been set," and changing them is a very long process. Therefore, Baker implored representatives from the FDA "to work with the controlled substances staff and FDA and with DEA . . . to allow for temporary increases in the manufacturing quota . . . so that when Manufacturer A has a problem, Manufacturers B, C, and D can temporarily step in."

Prohibiting pharmacies from transferring electronic prescriptions makes it more difficult to fill prescriptions without necessarily decreasing misuse, said Mahome. Indeed, she said, making prescribers send prescriptions to multiple pharmacies to find one that carries the prescribed medication can result in duplicate prescriptions. "Sometimes if the system does not automatically cancel the [prescription] that was sent, patients will go later and get that other prescription as well." She suggested that the DEA review this policy. Another area where the DEA might consider increasing oversight is in the issuing of controlled substance licenses, suggested Mahome. "Some providers should not be allowed to prescribe stimulants if they don't know how to do so effectively and do it well." She suggested requiring providers to answer questions about these drugs to receive a controlled substance license.

Starting with Nonstimulants

Given the problems of misuse and abuse associated with stimulant medications, Goodman suggested that nonstimulants be moved up in the armamentarium so that newly diagnosed patients would be started on a nonstimulant along with cognitive behavioral therapy and organizational techniques and move on from there. Starting patients on nonstimulants would be a very good idea, agreed Gordon, "because if that works, we'll stick with it forever." Even just choosing an extended-release formulation of a stimulant instead of an immediate-release formulation is "a simple thing that adult prescribers could do if appropriate for the patient," said Rubin, and could reduce the potential for misuse.

The old understanding of ADHD, which favors use of stimulants over nonstimulants, needs to change, said Arnsten. It is a mistake to focus on narrowing attention as a therapeutic effect, she said, which is based on old rating scales for stimulants. "Narrowing [of attention] is not always a good thing," she added. "It can interfere with creative pursuits, it can interfere with social interactions. [Let's] not narrow in on narrowing in," and instead emphasize self-regulation, which may be more conducive to prescribing nonstimulants.

The FDA has put a black box warning on all antidepressants to high-light the possible risk of suicidal thinking or behavior in young people, said Matthew Rudorfer, chief of the Psychopharmacology, Somatic, and Integrated Treatment Research Program at the National Institute of Mental Health, and this may discourage clinicians from trying new treatments such as viloxazine, an antidepressant nonstimulant that is now being marketed for treatment of ADHD (Edinoff et al., 2021). He suggested that the FDA revisit the warning on antidepressants regarding increasing suicidality, "because if that is discouraging otherwise appropriate use [for adult ADHD], it would be a fixable problem."

Untreated ADHD and Substance Use Disorder

McNeil highlighted "the extreme barriers to care that people experience across the life course" that can prevent them from being diagnosed with ADHD until late in life, if ever. These barriers are often shaped by structural racism and classism, he said, noting that untreated ADHD appears to underlie many individuals' long history of illicit stimulant use. To illustrate the possible relationship between untreated ADHD and SUD, McNeil cited the experiences of people who used illicit stimulants in Vancouver, Canada (McNeil et al., 2022). As a harm reduction measure during the COVID-19 epidemic, guidelines were changed to allow these individuals to receive prescription stimulants, "to provide an alternative in the context of a very toxic and volatile drug supply." McNeil found that many participants who received a stimulant prescription for the first time responded, "Oh my God, what is this, and why haven't I had access to this my entire life?" McNeil challenged participants to consider the "carceral logic" embedded in the language of "diversion," "misuse," and "abuse" that criminalizes people based on what they are using, "and really consider that it's use not as indicated, but it's often being done for medical reasons."

Harmful Use Is Not the Same as Abuse

"We are moving away from the word 'abuse,'" said Molina. "Abuse" places full responsibility on the individual "rather than recognizing the external factors that drive the use of substances" and that sometimes compel movement from use to uncontrolled use, she said. These external factors are present at multiple levels, from environmental and societal all the way down to interpersonal, and include stressors related to discrimination. Molina prefers the term "harmful use," although "misuse" is also employed.

Recreational misuse of stimulants to get high, experiment, or party longer occurs far less often than misuse to boost academic performance (Arria et al., 2008), said Molina. This trend contrasts starkly with pain medication, which is commonly misused to get high or to relieve pain. "We don't see that kind of thing with stimulants. . . . They are very, very different substances," she noted.

Stimulants are like electricity, suggested Blanco. The challenge is to use them effectively without being electrocuted. El-Sabawi pushed back on this. "Before we ask ourselves, 'How do we not get burned?'" she said, "we need to ask ourselves who is touching the socket and why." In particular, she noted that much of the research on ADHD is done on "White people, oftentimes White males, and we make policy recommendations based on the research . . . without understanding . . . if that study population is truly representative of the population that these policies are going to be impacting."

Diagnostic tools need to be developed with the broader population in mind, said El-Sabawi, not just white college-aged folks. ADHD does not look the same in everybody, she said. It looks different in women and people in color. There might be particular barriers for diagnosis of immigrants, and "we haven't talked about . . . how to make diagnosis and treatment more culturally sensitive. These are important conversations to have before we can talk about population-level regulatory changes or recommendations," she added.

It is incredibly important to "understand what the electricity [stimulant] is and what that means for you," said Seliby Perkins, a Black woman. "As an African American woman who's a descendant of slaves, there are some real things that this medical system has done to my people which make them very, very mistrusting," she noted. To build that trust, she uses shared decision making with all her patients so "they can educate me about what's holding them back."

Integrating a Concern for Stimulant Misuse into Clinical Assessments

Concerns about stimulant misuse should be addressed in the initial assessment of adults for ADHD, said Olfson. Often, he said, an individual seeking care fills out a self-report form to give the provider a sense of how severe their ADHD symptoms are. "That needs to be followed up with a [probing] clinical interview," he continued, to better understand the severity, timing, length, and persistence of the symptoms identified. The interview will also allow the clinician to learn how the patient's symptoms are affecting their life. Collateral information from relatives or coworkers can help document childhood onset and separate ADHD from other disorders, added Olfson, noting that "about half of adults with ADHD also have anxiety disorders [and] about a third have depression. . . . Separating out what is ADHD can be a difficult process." Neuropsychological assessments may also help, he said. Olfson, like others, emphasized the importance of impairment in diagnosing adult ADHD, noting that it is not just about the symptoms on the symptom checklists but about "how [symptoms] are interfering with adaptive functioning" in a patient's life. When evaluating impairment for people with ADHD, he said, "it's important to assess broadly . . . how the symptoms of impulsivity and hyperactivity and inattention are affecting their ability to form healthy, stable, romantic relationships," as well as the impact on friendships, work, parenting, and student achievement.

The evaluation should include a careful history of substance use, said Olfson, and this should be weighed in deciding whether to start a patient on a stimulant or nonstimulant medication. Noting that adults with ADHD are at increased risk for "motor vehicle accidents and other injuries, impulsive and risky sexual behavior, impulsive acts like shoplifting, and things like that," Olfson observed that ADHD can create "a whole cascade of problems for people in their lives, and it's important that we try to understand that and bring that into the clinical situation" to help people function better.

Training Physicians in Stimulant Diversion Prevention

The most common source of stimulants outside of a prescription is same-age peers with prescriptions for ADHD, which has implications for prevention, said Molina. However, she noted that nearly half of physician specialists surveyed in a recent study (Colaneri et al., 2018) felt inadequately qualified "to educate high-school-aged patients on the health risks and legal consequences of stimulant use and diversion."

To help address these concerns, Molina worked with practicing physicians and physician-scientists to develop usable strategies for preventing diversion of stimulants by patients. For this initial study, researchers recruited 114 18-to-25-year-old college students who were being treated with stimulants for ADHD (Colaneri et al., 2018; Molina et al., 2020). Of these, 17 percent reported that they had diverted their stimulants. Molina and colleagues developed a training package, trained the students' physicians, and reassessed the students. Although diversion was not significantly decreased by training, some risk factors decreased, including disclosure (letting others know that they had stimulants), the frequency with which they were approached to divert pills, and their intentions to divert pills.

To test the efficacy of physician training in preventing diversion, Molina and colleagues studied 341 13-to-18-year-olds in pediatric care in a total of 7 practices (McGuier et al., 2022). Following a baseline assessment, practices were randomly assigned to have all their providers trained or not. Noting that there is not a lot of stimulant diversion within this age group, Molina said, "this is a critical point in substance use prevention. You don't wait till the horse is out of the barn. . . . You try to do it preventively, proactively." At baseline, the researchers found that the older the children, the more likely they were to disclose their stimulant use and to be approached to share or sell their pills (Molina et al., 2021). They were also less likely to take their pills on a daily basis and thus were building up a supply that might create an opportunity for diversion. Older children were also more likely to have substance use problems and riskier peer environments (Molina et al., 2021).

Molina and colleagues developed a one-hour interactive stimulant diversion prevention (SDP) workshop for all physicians and staff in a pediatric care practice (McGuier et al., 2022). The SDP training boiled down to three essential points: 1) educate your patient, 2) be attentive to their supply of drugs, and 3) assess and manage their risk. Slides and video demonstrations offered providers advice for how to approach these tasks, with an emphasis on discussion and shared decision making. Physicians were given specific suggestions regarding patient and family education, medication management, assessment of mental health symptoms and functioning, and assessment of risky behavior.

In follow-up assessments (McGuier et al., 2022), the physicians who had been trained reported a change in patient-family education, which was "a pretty gratifying finding," said Molina. Physicians' attitudes regarding their ability to effect meaningful change also improved as a result of training. Molina noted that the trained physicians' increase in knowledge and skill was the most important driver toward changing their behavior. Longitudinal follow-ups of both pediatric and adult studies are in progress to see whether SDP training reduced diversion.

Regarding the larger goal of harm reduction, Molina cautioned that SDP is just one piece of the solution and that "tackling any type of substance use needs a multilayered approach." She also emphasized the importance of developing culturally sensitive approaches. "Ultimately," she said, "we really do need to think about beginning early" with developmentally appropriate approaches and not wait until adulthood to prevent stimulant diversion. As for training, in addition to communicating these messages through continuing education and patient education, Molina recommended teaching SDP in graduate school and residency programs.

LOOKING TOWARD THE FUTURE

Informing Policies and Practice

The effort to formulate sensible solutions to improve treatment for ADHD and reduce misuse must be based on a solid foundation of knowledge, said Arria. She suggested crafting a research agenda to establish this foundation, based on a three-level framework: 1) the clinical level, 2) the provider level, and 3) the systems level.

At the clinical level, longitudinal studies should seek to understand predictors of heterogeneity in the long-term trajectories of people with ADHD, said Arria. Some examples of potential predictors could be management of psychiatric comorbidity or aspects of young people's social and digital environments.

At the provider level, "we need a fuller understanding of the sources of information and misunderstanding that they have about ADHD," she said. Implementation science should be employed "to proactively track provider behavior as new guidelines are rolled out," to understand the facilitators and barriers to their adoption, and to identify which providers are "using an evidence-based mix of pharmacologic and nonpharmacologic strategies [and] collaborating with professionals . . . to maximize outcomes."

At the systems level, it is important to understand how policies and practices are influencing the delivery of care to people with ADHD, said Arria. This includes the actions of educational systems and employers; accrediting bodies; and local, state, and federal agencies. Arria noted that "the most potent improvements in population-based health come through policies and practice change." All research findings should be translated into "practical strategies to improve access to care and the lives of individuals with ADHD," she said.

Increasing Academic, Industry, and
Government Research on Adult ADHD

Goodman called NIH's annual $5.5 million expenditure on ADHD research "appalling. . . in 2023, with 20 years of growing international research." He said adult ADHD research funding needs to be increased to parity with child ADHD; "otherwise we are not moving the needle."

Diagnosis and treatment of ADHD in adults could be dramatically improved if a biomarker was available, said Farchione. "This is where the funding for research comes in. If we had a better understanding of the biology or more objective measures to use in clinical studies . . . it would be a game-changer," she said. Given the complexity and heterogeneity of ADHD is subjective by its very nature, Goodman was skeptical about finding an objective measure. However, he noted, it might be possible to combine genetic, molecular, and imaging markers, with the help of artificial intelligence tools, "to sort out the connectomes that are disrupted and the genetics that contribute to that."

Even if adult ADHD becomes widely recognized as a valid diagnosis, the relationship of risk to benefit of pharmacotherapy may be mismatched in people's beliefs, said Winterstein. To overcome this, she said, research needs to be able to quantify the likely benefits of treatment as well as severity and frequency of safety concerns for each patient.

What the field of adult ADHD really needs is "a true outcomes trial" to study interventions, comparable to MTA trial of pediatric ADHD (Swanson et al., 2008), said Baker. "I suspect, with a three-to-four-year period to compare treatment versus nontreatment of ADHD . . . we would see tremendous outcomes," he said. The impact of such a study, he said, could be comparable to that of the Scandinavian Simvastatin Survival Study trial, which showed that taking a statin to reduce cholesterol improved survival, thereby making a significant difference in the treatment of hypercholesterolemia (Pedersen et al., 2004). "There are twice as many adults with ADHD in the U.S. as kids," he added, so "it is really a long time coming."

Sokolowska noted the existence of data gaps even for treatments that have been FDA approved for certain populations and suggested that NIH and other organizations fill these gaps by extending the research to other populations and performing comparative evaluations of efficacy and risk. "We all would benefit from closing those gaps," she said. A workshop participant suggested that information on ADHD could be included when data is collected for school research, mental health surveys, or depression studies. Childress encouraged women with ADHD who are pregnant to sign up with the National Pregnancy Registry for Psychiatric Medications (MGH, 2008). Registering would enable follow-up to track adverse events, side effects, or other problems, and provide more information for women in the future, she said.

Targeted Drug Studies for Adult ADHD

Many speakers agreed that new medications are needed to treat adult ADHD but that a more practical first step would be better implementing existing treatments. Guanfacine, for example, seems to be "underutilized" in adults, for whom its use is off-label, said Rudorfer. Likewise, he said, data presented at this meeting suggest that initiation of any medicine should perhaps be accompanied by CBT. While there are no data to address that specific question, he said, existing medications "probably have not [been] fully optimized." ADHD should be treated more like depression, which has "so many different drugs," said Seliby Perkins. "We have to do better with the treatments we have, but also continue to look for better, newer treatments," she said.

"We need better ways to personalize treatment," said Rudorfer, but because each treatment was developed in isolation, it is a challenge to integrate them. The fact that only 8 percent of adults with ADHD are treated with nonstimulants raises questions of "who are those 8 percent, [and] are those the right 8 percent?" He suggested that the nonstimulants guanfacine and clonidine, which have been approved for children and adolescents with ADHD, and other medicines like buproprion and modafinil be tested in adults. Some of these gaps in knowledge are confounded by the way medications are approved, which leaves little interest in studying drugs that are no longer on patent, he noted.

"Most advances in medication in psychiatry have been by accident, even the stimulants . . . and then we worked backwards to try to figure out . . . how come they're working," noted Rudorfer. Newer brain research offers a translational approach and the possibility of developing a treatment to address a specific biochemical deficit. Rudorfer praised the National Institute of Mental Health's Research Domain Criteria initiative, which is "aimed at seeking pathology, especially in brain circuits, that might cut across diagnoses." Given the way certain ADHD symptoms are also present in depression and other conditions, he said, this could help researchers "learn from each other or form new collaborations." Rudorfer also suggested testing the external trigeminal nerve stimulation device, which was only approved for children with ADHD up to age 12, on older individuals (Loo et al., 2021).

Unlike the results of controlled clinical trials, "what we don't have," said Arria, is "a good understanding of providers in their natural habitat, what they do in their practice and what outcomes are resulting." She suggested funding a prospective study of new enrollees to various types of practices, collecting data on patient history and all treatments they are given, and monitoring outcomes over 5 to 10 years "to see what mix of strategies works for what kind of patients."

"We need more qualitative research . . . more observational research . . . [and] more researchers of color," said El-Sabawi. "We need to stop funding the same people over and over again and get some people who are new and . . . have . . . ties to the communities." El-Sabawi noted she is able to recruit people of color for her studies because she has spent years doing participatory action research and developing relationships with community groups. Seliby Perkins advocated for community-based participatory research, where "you can bring in a teacher, you can bring in the whole collaborative model; that is important." Lee suggested identifying the first provider that individuals would come in contact with and then "reverse engineer" to develop early detection and treatment models, using community-based participatory research methods.

Incentivizing Studies of Adults with ADHD

Drug development will need innovation to catch up with the need for approved medications to treat adults with ADHD, said Rudorfer, noting that clinical trials for attention deficit disorder medications in the 1990s did not include subjects over the age of 17. Given that FDA can only act on the data it receives, he suggested that perhaps incentives for industry, such as a longer patent clock, to conduct studies to expand drug labeling for adults may be appropriate.

Arnsten pointed to the value for incentives to pursue new mechanisms for drug development, such that new types of drugs rather than additional stimulant formulations would receive higher-value rewards. Any new drug would have to be affordable for managed care pharmacy, so one approach could be for companies to maintain exclusive rights for a long enough period of time to make it worth the cost of development. As of now, she said, "there is little motivation for a company to take on that kind of risk." An incentive that guarantees exclusivity for 10 years without competition from generics would require legislation. As an example, Lietzan pointed to the Generating Antibiotic Incentives Now Act, which was intended to spur innovation of new antibiotics by extending the exclusivity period for qualified infectious disease products. "The challenge will be making the case to policymakers," she said. A case could be made in terms of the broad social cost associated with the immediate-release psychostimulants and the long-term social benefit that could be derived from incentivizing these other products, she added.

References

ADDA (Attention Deficit Disorder Association). 2022. *Understanding ADHD*. https://add. org/adhd-in-adults/ (accessed March 2, 2024).

Adler, L. A., J. Adams, J. Madera-McDonough, E. Kohegyi, M. Hobart, D. Chang, M. Angelicola, R. McQuade, and M. Liebowitz. 2022. Efficacy, safety, and tolerability of centanafadine sustained-release tablets in adults with attention-deficit/hyperactivity disorder: Results of 2 Phase 3, randomized, double-blind, multicenter, placebo-controlled trials. *J Clin Psychopharmacol* 42(5):429-439.

Adler, L. A., S. V. Faraone, T. J. Spencer, P. Berglund, S. Alperin, and R. C. Kessler. 2017. The structure of adult ADHD. *Int J Methods Psychiatr Res* 26(1).

Advokat, C. D., D. Guidry, and L. Martino. 2008. Licit and illicit use of medications for attention-deficit hyperactivity disorder in undergraduate college students. *J Am Coll Health* 56(6):601-606.

Akili Interactive Labs. 2024. *EndeavorOTC*. https://www.endeavorotc.com/ (accessed March 5, 2024.

Aluri, J., D. Goodman, K. Antshel, and R. Mojtabai. 2023. Variation in ADHD treatment by mental health care setting among us college students from 2019 to 2022. *J Atten Disord* 27(12):1411-1419.

APA (American Psychiatric Association). 2013. *Diagnostic and statistical manual of mental disorders (5th ed.)*. Washington, DC: American Psychiatric Publishing. https://psycnet. apa.org/record/2013-14907-000 (accessed April 29, 2024).

Arcos-Burgos, M., and M. T. Acosta. 2007. Tuning major gene variants conditioning human behavior: The anachronism of ADHD. *Curr Opin Genet Dev* 17(3):234-238.

Ariely, D. 2023. *Misbelief: What makes rational people believe irrational things*. New York: HarperCollins.

Arnsten, A. F., and S. R. Pliszka. 2011. Catecholamine influences on prefrontal cortical function: Relevance to treatment of attention deficit/hyperactivity disorder and related disorders. *Pharmacol Biochem Behav* 99(2):211-216.

Arnsten, A. F. T., and M. Wang. 2020. The evolutionary expansion of mGluR3-NAAG-GCPII signaling: Relevance to human intelligence and cognitive disorders. *Am J Psychiatry* 177(12):1103-1106.

Arria, A. M., K. M. Caldeira, K. E. O'Grady, K. B. Vincent, E. P. Johnson, and E. D. Wish. 2008. Nonmedical use of prescription stimulants among college students: Associations with attention-deficit-hyperactivity disorder and polydrug use. *Pharmacotherapy* 28(2):156-169.

Arria, A. M., K. M. Caldeira, K. B. Vincent, K. E. O'Grady, M. D. Cimini, I. M. Geisner, N. Fossos-Wong, J. R. Kilmer, and M. E. Larimer. 2017. Do college students improve their grades by using prescription stimulants nonmedically? *Addict Behav* 65:245-249.

Arrondo, G., M. Mulraney, I. Iturmendi-Sabater, H. Musullulu, L. Gambra, T. Niculcea, T. Banaschewski, E. Simonoff, M. Döpfner, S. P. Hinshaw, D. Coghill, and S. Cortese. 2024. Systematic review and meta-analysis: Clinical utility of continuous performance tests for the identification of attention-deficit/hyperactivity disorder. *J Am Acad Child Adolesc Psychiatry* 63(2):154-171.

Asherson, P., and H. Gurling. 2011. Quantitative and molecular genetics of ADHD. In *Behavioral neuroscience of attention deficit hyperactivity disorder and its treatment.* Vol. 9, Current topics in behavioral neurosciences, edited by C. Stanford and R. Tannock. Berlin, Heidelberg: Springer.

Attention Deficit Disorder Association. 2022. *Understanding ADHD.* https://add.org/adhd-in-adults (accessed March 2, 2024).

Barkley, R. A., and M. Fischer. 2019. Hyperactive child syndrome and estimated life expectancy at young adult follow-up: The role of ADHD persistence and other potential predictors. *J Atten Disord* 23(9):907-923.

Bauer, A. M., M. M. Parker, D. Schillinger, W. Katon, N. Adler, A. S. Adams, H. H. Moffet, and A. J. Karter. 2014. Associations between antidepressant adherence and shared decision-making, patient–provider trust, and communication among adults with diabetes: Diabetes study of Northern California (distance). *Journal of General Internal Medicine* 29(8):1139-1147.

Bejerot, S., E. M. Rydén, and C. M. Arlinde. 2010. Two-year outcome of treatment with central stimulant medication in adult attention-deficit/hyperactivity disorder: A prospective study. *J Clin Psychiatry* 71(12):1590-1597.

Benson, K., K. Flory, K. L. Humphreys, and S. S. Lee. 2015. Misuse of stimulant medication among college students: A comprehensive review and meta-analysis. *Clin Child Fam Psychol Rev* 18(1):50-76.

Bernardina Dalla, M. D., C. O. Ayala, F. Cristina de Abreu Quintela Castro, F. K. Neto, G. Zanirati, W. Cañon-Montañez, and R. Mattiello. 2022. Environmental pollution and attention deficit hyperactivity disorder: A meta-analysis of cohort studies. *Environ Pollut* 315:120351.

Berridge, C. W., D. M. Devilbiss, M. E. Andrzejewski, A. F. Arnsten, A. E. Kelley, B. Schmeichel, C. Hamilton, and R. C. Spencer. 2006. Methylphenidate preferentially increases catecholamine neurotransmission within the prefrontal cortex at low doses that enhance cognitive function. *Biol Psychiatry* 60(10):1111-1120.

Berridge, C. W., and R. C. Spencer. 2016. Differential cognitive actions of norepinephrine $\alpha2$ and $\alpha1$ receptor signaling in the prefrontal cortex. *Brain Res* 1641(Pt B):189-196.

Bowman, E., D. Coghill, C. Murawski, and P. Bossaerts. 2023. Not so smart? "Smart" drugs increase the level but decrease the quality of cognitive effort. *Sci Adv* 9(24):eadd4165.

Brod, M., J. Johnston, S. Able, and R. Swindle. 2006. Validation of the adult attention-deficit/hyperactivity disorder quality-of-life scale (AAQoL): A disease-specific quality-of-life measure. *Qual Life Res* 15(1):117-129.

Brown, N. M., S. N. Brown, R. D. Briggs, M. Germán, P. F. Belamarich, and S. O. Oyeku. 2017. Associations between adverse childhood experiences and ADHD diagnosis and severity. *Acad Pediatr* 17(4):349-355.

Burgard, D. A., R. Fuller, B. Becker, R. Ferrell, and M. J. Dinglasan-Panlilio. 2013. Potential trends in attention deficit hyperactivity disorder (ADHD) drug use on a college campus: Wastewater analysis of amphetamine and ritalinic acid. *Sci Total Environ* 450-451:242-249.

Callen, E. F., T. L. Clay, J. Alai, D. W. Goodman, L. A. Adler, J. Shields, and S. V. Faraone. 2023. Progress and pitfalls in the provision of quality care for adults with attention deficit hyperactivity disorder in primary care. *J Atten Disord* 27(6):575-582.

Canadian ADHD Resource Alliance (CADDRA). 2020. Canadian ADHD practice guidelines, 4.1 edition, Toronto ON; CADDRA, 2020. https://adhdlearn.caddra.ca/purchase-guidelines/ (accessed April 29, 2024).

Cassidy, T. A., E. C. McNaughton, S. Varughese, L. Russo, M. Zulueta, and S. F. Butler. 2015. Nonmedical use of prescription ADHD stimulant medications among adults in a substance abuse treatment population: Early findings from the NAVIPPRO surveillance system. *J Atten Disord* 19(4):275-283.

CHADD (Children and Adults with ADHD). 2023. ADHD medications approved by the US Food and Drug Administration.

Chamberlain, S. R., S. Cortese, and J. E. Grant. 2021. Screening for adult ADHD using brief rating tools: What can we conclude from a positive screen? Some caveats. *Compr Psychiatry* 106:152224.

Chang, Z., L. Ghirardi, P. D. Quinn, P. Asherson, B. M. D'Onofrio, and H. Larsson. 2019. Risks and benefits of attention-deficit/hyperactivity disorder medication on behavioral and neuropsychiatric outcomes: A qualitative review of pharmacoepidemiology studies using linked prescription databases. *Biol Psychiatry* 86(5):335-343.

Chang, Z., P. Lichtenstein, L. Halldner, B. D'Onofrio, E. Serlachius, S. Fazel, N. Långström, and H. Larsson. 2014. Stimulant ADHD medication and risk for substance abuse. *J Child Psychol Psychiatry* 55(8):878-885.

Cherkasova, M. V., A. Roy, B. S. G. Molina, G. Scott, G. Weiss, R. A. Barkley, J. Biederman, M. Uchida, S. P. Hinshaw, E. B. Owens, and L. Hechtman. 2022. Review: Adult outcome as seen through controlled prospective follow-up studies of children with attention-deficit/hyperactivity disorder followed into adulthood. *J Am Acad Child Adolesc Psychiatry* 61(3):378-391.

Childress, A. and G. W. Mattingly. 2023. Assessing practice patterns in care of adults with ADHD. online: Medscape. https://www.medscape.org/viewarticle/998074 (accessed April 29, 2024).

Chung, W., S. F. Jiang, D. Paksarian, A. Nikolaidis, F. X. Castellanos, K. R. Merikangas, and M. P. Milham. 2019. Trends in the prevalence and incidence of attention-deficit/hyperactivity disorder among adults and children of different racial and ethnic groups. *JAMA Netw Open* 2(11):e1914344.

Clark, S. V., T. D. Satterthwaite, T. Z. King, R. D. Morris, E. Zendehrouh, and J. A. Turner. 2022. Cerebellum-cingulo-opercular network connectivity strengthens in adolescence and supports attention efficiency only in childhood. *Dev Cogn Neurosci* 56:101129.

Clever, S. L., D. E. Ford, L. V. Rubenstein, K. M. Rost, L. S. Meredith, C. D. Sherbourne, N.-Y. Wang, J. J. Arbelaez, and L. A. Cooper. 2006. Primary care patients' involvement in decision-making is associated with improvement in depression. *Medical Care* 44(5):398-405.

CMS (Centers for Medicare & Medicaid Services). 2016. *Drug diversion: What is a prescriber's role in preventing the diversion of prescription drugs?* https://www.hhs.gov/guidance/sites/default/files/hhs-guidance-documents/DrugDiversionFS022316.pdf (accessed April 29, 2024).

Colaneri, N., S. A. Keim, and A. Adesman. 2018. Physician training and qualification to educate patients on attention-deficit/hyperactivity disorder stimulant diversion and misuse. *J Child Adolesc Psychopharmacol* 28(8):554-561.

Connolly, J. J., J. T. Glessner, J. Elia, and H. Hakonarson. 2015. ADHD & pharmacotherapy: Past, present, and future: A review of the changing landscape of drug therapy for attention deficit hyperactivity disorder. *Ther Innov Regul Sci* 49(5):632-642.

Cools, R., and A. F. T. Arnsten. 2022. Neuromodulation of prefrontal cortex cognitive function in primates: The powerful roles of monoamines and acetylcholine. *Neuropsychopharmacology* 47(1):309-328.

Cortese, S., N. Adamo, C. Del Giovane, C. Mohr-Jensen, A. J. Hayes, S. Carucci, L. Z. Atkinson, L. Tessari, T. Banaschewski, D. Coghill, C. Hollis, E. Simonoff, A. Zuddas, C. Barbui, M. Purgato, H. C. Steinhausen, F. Shokraneh, J. Xia, and A. Cipriani. 2018. Comparative efficacy and tolerability of medications for attention-deficit hyperactivity disorder in children, adolescents, and adults: A systematic review and network meta-analysis. *Lancet Psychiatry* 5(9):727-738.

Cortese, S., and C. Fava. 2024. Long-term cardiovascular effects of medications for attention-deficit/hyperactivity disorder-balancing benefits and risks of treatment. *JAMA Psychiatry* 81(2):123-124.

Cortese, S., M. Song, L. C. Farhat, D. K. Yon, S. W. Lee, M. S. Kim, S. Park, J. W. Oh, S. Lee, K. A. Cheon, L. Smith, C. J. Gosling, G. V. Polanczyk, H. Larsson, L. A. Rohde, S. V. Faraone, A. Koyanagi, E. Dragioti, J. Radua, A. F. Carvalho, J. Il Shin, and M. Solmi. 2023. Incidence, prevalence, and global burden of ADHD from 1990 to 2019 across 204 countries: Data, with critical re-analysis, from the global burden of disease study. *Mol Psychiatry* 28(11):4823-4830.

Crump, C., J. Sundquist, and K. Sundquist. 2023. Preterm or early term birth and risk of attention-deficit/hyperactivity disorder: A national cohort and co-sibling study. *Ann Epidemiol* 86:119-125.e114.

Danielson, M. L., M. K. Bohm, K. Newsome, A. H. Claussen, J. W. Kaminski, S. D. Grosse, L. Siwakoti, A. Arifkhanova, R. H. Bitsko, and L. R. Robinson. 2023. Trends in stimulant prescription fills among commercially insured children and adults—United States, 2016-2021. *MMWR Morb Mortal Wkly Rep* 72(13):327-332.

DeSantis, A., S. M. Noar, and E. M. Webb. 2010. Speeding through the frat house: A qualitative exploration of nonmedical adhd stimulant use in fraternities. *J Drug Educ* 40(2):157-171.

DeSantis, A. D., and A. C. Hane. 2010. "Adderall is definitely not a drug": Justifications for the illegal use of ADHD stimulants. *Subst Use Misuse* 45(1-2):31-46.

Edinoff, A. N., H. A. Akuly, J. H. Wagner, M. A. Boudreaux, L. A. Kaplan, S. Yusuf, E. E. Neuchat, E. M. Cornett, A. G. Boyer, A. M. Kaye, and A. D. Kaye. 2021. Viloxazine in the treatment of attention deficit hyperactivity disorder. *Front Psychiatry* 12:789982.

Fairman, K. A., A. M. Peckham, and D. A. Sclar. 2020. Diagnosis and treatment of ADHD in the United States: Update by gender and race. *Journal of Attention Disorders* 24(1):10-19.

Faraone, S. V., M. A. Bellgrove, I. Brikell, S. Cortese, C. A. Hartman, C. Hollis, J. H. Newcorn, A. Philipsen, G. V. Polanczyk, K. Rubia, M. H. Sibley, and J. K. Buitelaar. 2024. Attention-deficit/hyperactivity disorder. *Nat Rev Dis Primers* 10(1):11.

Faraone, S. V., A. L. Rostain, C. B. Montano, O. Mason, K. M. Antshel, and J. H. Newcorn. 2020. Systematic review: Nonmedical use of prescription stimulants: Risk factors, outcomes, and risk reduction strategies. *J Am Acad Child Adolesc Psychiatry* 59(1):100-112.

FDA (U.S. Food and Drug Adminstration). 2017. *Assessment of abuse potential of drugs.* FDA-2010-D-0026. https://www.fda.gov/regulatory-information/search-fda-guidance-documents/assessment-abuse-potential-drugs (accessed April 29, 2024).

FDA. 2019. *Attention deficit hyperactivity disorder: Developing stimulant drugs for treatment guidance for industry*. FDA-2019-D-0849. https://www.fda.gov/regulatory-information/search-fda-guidance-documents/attention-deficit-hyperactivity-disorder-developing-stimulant-drugs-treatment-guidance-industry (accessed April 29, 2024).

FDA. 2022. *FDA announces shortage of Adderall*. https://www.fda.gov/drugs/drug-safety-and-availability/fda-announces-shortage-adderall (accessed April 29, 2024).

FDA. 2023a. *FDA updating warnings to improve safe use of prescription stimulants used to treat adhd and other conditions*. https://www.fda.gov/drugs/drug-safety-and-availability/fda-updating-warnings-improve-safe-use-prescription-stimulants-used-treat-adhd-and-other-conditions (accessed March 24, 2024).

FDA. 2023b. *Treating and dealing with ADHD*. https://www.fda.gov/consumers/consumer-updates/treating-and-dealing-adhd#:~:text=The%20FDA%20has%20also%20approved,be%20best%20for%20your%20child. (accessed March 24, 2024).

FDA. n.d. *Overview of the 505(b)(2) regulatory pathway for new drug applications* https://www.fda.gov/media/156350/download.

FDA and DEA (U.S. Food and Drug Adminstration and U.S. Drug and Enforcement Agency). 2023. *Joint letter: Updating on the ongoing prescription stimulant shortages* https://www.fda.gov/media/170736/download?attachment

Findling, R. L. 2008. Evolution of the treatment of attention-deficit/hyperactivity disorder in children: A review. *Clin Ther* 30(5):942-957.

Fredriksson, I., N. Jayaram-Lindström, M. Wirf, E. Nylander, E. Nyström, K. Jardemark, and P. Steensland. 2015. Evaluation of guanfacine as a potential medication for alcohol use disorder in long-term drinking rats: Behavioral and electrophysiological findings. *Neuropsychopharmacology* 40(5):1130-1140.

Galvin, V. C., A. F. T. Arnsten, and M. Wang. 2020. Involvement of nicotinic receptors in working memory function. *Curr Top Behav Neurosci* 45:89-99.

Gerhard, T., A. G. Winterstein, M. Olfson, C. Huang, A. Saidi, and S. Crystal. 2010. Pre-existing cardiovascular conditions and pharmacological treatment of adult ADHD. *Pharmacoepidemiology and Drug Safety* 19(5):457-464.

Goodman, D. 2023. ASPARD development of clinical practice guidelines for the diagnosis and treatment for ADHD in adults. online: ASPARD.

Goodman, D. W., and G. Mattingly. 2023. Practice guidelines development: The ASPARD United States guidelines for the diagnosis and treatment of ADHD in adults. *Psychiatric Annals* 53(10):449-454.

Groom, M. J., and S. Cortese. 2022. Current pharmacological treatments for ADHD. *Curr Top Behav Neurosci* 57:19-50.

Hains, A. B., Y. Yabe, and A. F. Arnsten. 2015. Chronic stimulation of alpha-2α-adrenoceptors with guanfacine protects rodent prefrontal cortex dendritic spines and cognition from the effects of chronic stress. *Neurobiol Stress* 2:1-9.

Heal, D. J., S. L. Smith, J. Gosden, and D. J. Nutt. 2013. Amphetamine, past and present—a pharmacological and clinical perspective. *J Psychopharmacol* 27(6):479-496.

Hennissen, L., M. J. Bakker, T. Banaschewski, S. Carucci, D. Coghill, M. Danckaerts, R. W. Dittmann, C. Hollis, H. Kovshoff, S. McCarthy, P. Nagy, E. Sonuga-Barke, I. C. Wong, A. Zuddas, E. Rosenthal, and J. K. Buitelaar. 2017. Cardiovascular effects of stimulant and non-stimulant medication for children and adolescents with adhd: A systematic review and meta-analysis of trials of methylphenidate, amphetamines and atomoxetine. *CNS Drugs* 31(3):199-215.

HMP Global. n.d. *Psych congress*. https://www.hmpglobalevents.com/psych-congress (accessed March 5, 2024).

Hughes, A., M. R. Williams, R. N. Lipari, J. Bose, E. A. P. Copello, and L. A. Kroutil. 2016. Prescription drug use and misuse in the United States: Results from the 2015 National Survey on Drug Use and Health: NSDUH Data Review.

Humphreys, K. L., T. Eng, and S. S. Lee. 2013. Stimulant medication and substance use outcomes: A meta-analysis. *JAMA Psychiatry* 70(7):740-749.

Hupalo, S., and C. W. Berridge. 2016. Working memory impairing actions of corticotropin-releasing factor (CRF) neurotransmission in the prefrontal cortex. *Neuropsychopharmacology* 41(11):2733-2740.

Hupalo, S., A. J. Martin, R. K. Green, D. M. Devilbiss, and C. W. Berridge. 2019. Prefrontal corticotropin-releasing factor (CRF) neurons act locally to modulate frontostriatal cognition and circuit function. *J Neurosci* 39(11):2080-2090.

Hupalo, S., R. C. Spencer, and C. W. Berridge. 2021. Prefrontal corticotropin-releasing factor neurons impair sustained attention via distal transmitter release. *Eur J Neurosci*.

IQVIA (IQVIA Government Solutions). 2023. *Stimulant prescription trends in the United States from 2012-2022*. Falls Church, VA.

Iwanami, A., K. Saito, M. Fujiwara, D. Okutsu, and H. Ichikawa. 2020. Efficacy and safety of guanfacine extended-release in the treatment of attention-deficit/hyperactivity disorder in adults: Results of a randomized, double-blind, placebo-controlled study. *J Clin Psychiatry* 81(3).

Jean, F. A. M., J. Arsandaux, I. Montagni, O. Collet, M. Fatséas, M. Auriacombe, J. A. Ramos-Quiroga, S. M. Côté, C. Tzourio, and C. Galéra. 2022. Attention deficit hyperactivity disorder symptoms and cannabis use after one year among students of the i-Share cohort. *Eur Psychiatry* 65(1):1-18.

Kantak, K. M., and L. P. Dwoskin. 2016. Necessity for research directed at stimulant type and treatment-onset age to access the impact of medication on drug abuse vulnerability in teenagers with ADHD. *Pharmacol Biochem Behav* 145:24-26.

Kessler, R. 2006. The prevalence and correlates of adult adhd in the united states: Results from the national comorbidity survey replication. *American Journal of Psychiatry* 163(4).

Kilmer, J. R., N. Fossos-Wong, I. M. Geisner, J. C. Yeh, M. E. Larimer, M. D. Cimini, K. B. Vincent, H. K. Allen, L. A. Barrall, and A. M. Arria. 2021. Nonmedical use of prescription stimulants as a "red flag" for other substance use. *Subst Use Misuse* 56(7):941-949.

Kim, J. H., J. Y. Kim, J. Lee, G. H. Jeong, E. Lee, S. Lee, K. H. Lee, A. Kronbichler, B. Stubbs, M. Solmi, A. Koyanagi, S. H. Hong, E. Dragioti, L. Jacob, A. R. Brunoni, A. F. Carvalho, J. Radua, T. Thompson, L. Smith, H. Oh, L. Yang, I. Grabovac, F. Schuch, M. Fornaro, A. Stickley, T. B. Rais, G. Salazar de Pablo, J. I. Shin, and P. Fusar-Poli. 2020. Environmental risk factors, protective factors, and peripheral biomarkers for ADHD: An umbrella review. *Lancet Psychiatry* 7(11):955-970.

Kooij, S. J., S. Bejerot, A. Blackwell, H. Caci, M. Casas-Brugué, P. J. Carpentier, D. Edvinsson, J. Fayyad, K. Foeken, M. Fitzgerald, V. Gaillac, Y. Ginsberg, C. Henry, J. Krause, M. B. Lensing, I. Manor, H. Niederhofer, C. Nunes-Filipe, M. D. Ohlmeier, P. Oswald, S. Pallanti, A. Pehlivanidis, J. A. Ramos-Quiroga, M. Rastam, D. Ryffel-Rawak, S. Stes, and P. Asherson. 2010. European consensus statement on diagnosis and treatment of adult ADHD: The European network adult ADHD. *BMC Psychiatry* 10:67.

Kubik, J. A. 2010. Efficacy of ADHD coaching for adults with ADHD. *J Atten Disord* 13(5):442-453.

Lange, K. W., S. Reichl, K. M. Lange, L. Tucha, and O. Tucha. 2010. The history of attention deficit hyperactivity disorder. *Atten Defic Hyperact Disord* 2(4):241-255.

Larsson, H., Z. Chang, B. M. D'Onofrio, and P. Lichtenstein. 2014. The heritability of clinically diagnosed attention deficit hyperactivity disorder across the lifespan. *Psychol Med* 44(10):2223-2229.

Lee, S. M., H. K. Cheong, I. H. Oh, and M. Hong. 2021. Nationwide rate of adult ADHD diagnosis and pharmacotherapy from 2015 to 2018. *Int J Environ Res Public Health* 18(21).

Leffa, D. T., A. Caye, and L. A. Rohde. 2022. ADHD in children and adults: Diagnosis and prognosis. *Curr Top Behav Neurosci* 57:1-18.

Leib, S. I., R. D. Keezer, B. M. Cerny, L. R. Holbrook, V. T. Gallagher, K. J. Jennette, G. P. Ovsiew, and J. R. Soble. 2021. Distinct latent profiles of working memory and processing speed in adults with ADHD. *Dev Neuropsychol* 46(8):574-587.

Levine, S. Z., A. Rotstein, A. Kodesh, S. Sandin, B. K. Lee, G. Weinstein, M. Schnaider Beeri, and A. Reichenberg. 2023. Adult attention-deficit/hyperactivity disorder and the risk of dementia. *JAMA Netw Open* 6(10):e2338088.

Linssen, A. M., A. Sambeth, E. F. Vuurman, and W. J. Riedel. 2014. Cognitive effects of methylphenidate in healthy volunteers: A review of single dose studies. *Int J Neuropsychopharmacol* 17(6):961-977.

Liu, C. I., M. H. Hua, M. L. Lu, and K. K. Goh. 2023. Effectiveness of cognitive behavioural-based interventions for adults with attention-deficit/hyperactivity disorder extends beyond core symptoms: A meta-analysis of randomized controlled trials. *Psychol Psychother* 96(3):543-559.

Loo, S. K., G. C. Salgari, A. Ellis, J. Cowen, A. Dillon, and J. J. McGough. 2021. Trigeminal nerve stimulation for attention-deficit/hyperactivity disorder: Cognitive and electroencephalographic predictors of treatment response. *J Am Acad Child Adolesc Psychiatry* 60(7):856-864.e851.

Lopez, P. L., F. M. Torrente, A. Ciapponi, A. G. Lischinsky, M. Cetkovich-Bakmas, J. I. Rojas, M. Romano, and F. F. Manes. 2018. Cognitive-behavioural interventions for attention deficit hyperactivity disorder (ADHD) in adults. *Cochrane Database Syst Rev* 3(3):Cd010840.

Mattingly, T. J., II, D. A. Hyman, and G. Bai. 2023. Pharmacy benefit managers: History, business practices, economics, and policy. *JAMA Health Forum* 4(11):e233804-e233804.

May, T., E. Birch, K. Chaves, N. Cranswick, E. Culnane, J. Delaney, M. Derrick, V. Eapen, C. Edlington, D. Efron, T. Ewais, I. Garner, M. Gathercole, K. Jagadheesan, L. Jobson, J. Kramer, M. Mack, M. Misso, C. Murrup-Stewart, E. Savage, E. Sciberras, B. Singh, R. Testa, L. Vale, A. Weirman, E. Petch, K. Williams, and M. Bellgrove. 2023. The Australian evidence-based clinical practice guideline for attention deficit hyperactivity disorder. *Aust N Z J Psychiatry* 57(8):1101-1116.

McCabe, S. E., J. E. Schulenberg, T. S. Schepis, R. J. Evans-Polce, T. E. Wilens, V. V. McCabe, and P. T. Veliz. 2022. Trajectories of prescription drug misuse among us adults from ages 18 to 50 years. *JAMA Netw Open* 5(1):e2141995.

McCabe, S. E., J. E. Schulenberg, T. E. Wilens, T. S. Schepis, V. V. McCabe, and P. T. Veliz. 2023. Prescription stimulant medical and nonmedical use among us secondary school students, 2005 to 2020. *JAMA Netw Open* 6(4):e238707.

McGuier, E. A., D. J. Kolko, S. L. Pedersen, H. L. Kipp, H. M. Joseph, R. A. Lindstrom, D. J. Bauer, G. A. Subramaniam, and B. S. G. Molina. 2022. Effects of training on use of stimulant diversion prevention strategies by pediatric primary care providers: Results from a cluster-randomized trial. *Prev Sci* 23(7):1299-1307.

McNeil, R., T. Fleming, S. Mayer, A. Barker, M. Mansoor, A. Betsos, T. Austin, S. Parusel, A. Ivsins, and J. Boyd. 2022. Implementation of safe supply alternatives during intersecting COVID-19 and overdose health emergencies in British Columbia, Canada, 2021. *Am J Public Health* 112(S2):S151-s158.

MGH (Massachusetts General Hospital). 2008. *National pregnancy registry for psychiatric medications.* https://womensmentalhealth.org/research/pregnancyregistry/ (accessed April 30, 2024).

Michelini, G., A. Lenartowicz, J. P. Diaz-Fong, R. M. Bilder, J. J. McGough, J. T. McCracken, and S. K. Loo. 2023. Methylphenidate, guanfacine, and combined treatment effects on electroencephalography correlates of spatial working memory in attention-deficit/hyperactivity disorder. *J Am Acad Child Adolesc Psychiatry* 62(1):37-47.

Michielsen, M., E. Semeijn, H. C. Comijs, P. van de Ven, A. T. Beekman, D. J. Deeg, and J. J. Kooij. 2012. Prevalence of attention-deficit hyperactivity disorder in older adults in The Netherlands. *Br J Psychiatry* 201(4):298-305.

Molina, B. S., S. P. Hinshaw, L. Eugene Arnold, J. M. Swanson, W. E. Pelham, L. Hechtman, B. Hoza, J. N. Epstein, T. Wigal, H. B. Abikoff, L. L. Greenhill, P. S. Jensen, K. C. Wells, B. Vitiello, R. D. Gibbons, A. Howard, P. R. Houck, K. Hur, B. Lu, and S. Marcus. 2013. Adolescent substance use in the multimodal treatment study of attention-deficit/hyperactivity disorder (ADHD) (MTA) as a function of childhood ADHD, random assignment to childhood treatments, and subsequent medication. *J Am Acad Child Adolesc Psychiatry* 52(3):250-263.

Molina, B. S. G., H. M. Joseph, H. L. Kipp, R. A. Lindstrom, S. L. Pedersen, D. J. Kolko, D. J. Bauer, and G. A. Subramaniam. 2021. Adolescents treated for attention-deficit/hyperactivity disorder in pediatric primary care: Characterizing risk for stimulant diversion. *J Dev Behav Pediatr* 42(7):540-552.

Molina, B. S. G., T. M. Kennedy, A. L. Howard, J. M. Swanson, L. E. Arnold, J. T. Mitchell, A. Stehli, E. H. Kennedy, J. N. Epstein, L. T. Hechtman, S. P. Hinshaw, and B. Vitiello. 2023. Association between stimulant treatment and substance use through adolescence into early adulthood. *JAMA Psychiatry* 80(9):933-941.

Molina, B. S. G., H. L. Kipp, H. M. Joseph, S. A. Engster, S. C. Harty, M. Dawkins, R. A. Lindstrom, D. J. Bauer, and S. S. Bangalore. 2020. Stimulant diversion risk among college students treated for ADHD: Primary care provider prevention training. *Acad Pediatr* 20(1):119-127.

The MTA Cooperative Group. 1999. A 14-month randomized clinical trial of treatment strategies for attention-deficit/hyperactivity disorder. *Arch Gen Psychiatry* 56(12):1073-1086.

Mustonen, A., A. E. Alakokkare, J. G. Scott, A. H. Halt, M. Vuori, T. Hurtig, A. Rodriguez, J. Miettunen, and S. Niemelä. 2023. Association of ADHD symptoms in adolescence and mortality in northern Finland birth cohort 1986. *Nord J Psychiatry* 77(2):165-171.

Nasser, A., J. T. Hull, S. A. Chaturvedi, T. Liranso, O. Odebo, A. R. Kosheleff, N. Fry, A. J. Cutler, J. Rubin, S. Schwabe, and A. Childress. 2022. A Phase III, randomized, double-blind, placebo-controlled trial assessing the efficacy and safety of viloxazine extended-release capsules in adults with attention-deficit/hyperactivity disorder. *CNS Drugs* 36(8):897-915.

NAMI (National Alliance on Mental Illness). 2023. *Mental health by the numbers.* https://www.nami.org/about-mental-illness/mental-health-by-the-numbers/ (accessed April 26, 2024).

NCHS (National Center for Health Statistics). 2019. *National health interview survey.* https://www.cdc.gov/nchs/nhis/index.htm (accessed April 30, 2024).

NeuroSigma. 2022. *What is Monarch eTNS?* https://www.monarch-etns.com/ (accessed March 5, 2024).

NICE (National Institue for Health and Care Excellence, UK). 2018. *Attention deficit hyperactivity disorder: Diagnosis and management.* https://www.nice.org.uk/guidance/ng87 (accessed April 30, 2024).

NIH (National Institues of Health). 1998. Diagnosis and treatment of attention deficit hyperactivity disorder (ADHD). *NIH Consens Statement* 16(2):1-37.

Novak, S. P., L. A. Kroutil, R. L. Williams, and D. L. Van Brunt. 2007. The nonmedical use of prescription adhd medications: Results from a national internet panel. *Subst Abuse Treat Prev Policy* 2:32.

Office of the Surgeon General. 2021. Publications and reports of the Surgeon General. In *Confronting health misinformation: The U.S. Surgeon General's advisory on building a healthy information environment.* Washington (DC): Department of Health and Human Services.

Öhlund, L., M. Ott, R. Lundqvist, M. Sandlund, E. Salander Renberg, and U. Werneke. 2020. Suicidal and non-suicidal self-injurious behaviour in patients with bipolar disorder and comorbid attention deficit hyperactivity disorder after initiation of central stimulant treatment: A mirror-image study based on the LiSIE retrospective cohort. *Ther Adv Psychopharmacol* 10:2045125320947502.

Otsuka (Otsuka Pharmaceutical Development & Commercialization). 2022a. A trial of centanafadine efficacy and safety in adolescents with attention-deficit/hyperactivity disorder: Otsuka Pharmaceutical Development & Commercialization, Inc. Original edition, NCT05257265.

Otsuka. 2022b. A trial of centanafadine efficacy and safety in children with ADHD: Otsuka Pharmaceutical Development & Commercialization, Inc. Original edition, NCT05428033.

Pauly, V., E. Frauger, M. Lepelley, M. Mallaret, Q. Boucherie, and J. Micallef. 2018. Patterns and profiles of methylphenidate use both in children and adults. *Br J Clin Pharmacol* 84(6):1215-1227.

Pedersen, T. R., J. Kjekshus, K. Berg, T. Haghfelt, O. Faergeman, G. Faergeman, K. Pyörälä, T. Miettinen, L. Wilhelmsen, A. G. Olsson, and H. Wedel. 2004. Randomised trial of cholesterol lowering in 4444 patients with coronary heart disease: The Scandinavian simvastatin survival study (4s). 1994. *Atheroscler Suppl* 5(3):81-87.

Pehlivanidis, A., K. Papanikolaou, V. Mantas, E. Kalantzi, K. Korobili, L. A. Xenaki, G. Vassiliou, and C. Papageorgiou. 2020. Lifetime co-occurring psychiatric disorders in newly diagnosed adults with attention deficit hyperactivity disorder (ADHD) or/and autism spectrum disorder (ASD). *BMC Psychiatry* 20(1):423.

Phillips, E. L., and A. E. McDaniel. 2018. *College prescription drug study key findings report.* Center for the Study of Student Life, Columbus, Ohio: The Ohio State University.

Pohl, J., P. Pittman, M. Anslie, M. B. Bigley, and T. Kopanos. A decade of data: An update on the primary care and mental health nurse practitioner and physician workforce. *Health Affairs.*

Pujol-Gualdo, N., C. Sanchez-Mora, J. A. Ramos-Quiroga, M. Ribases, and M. Soler Artigas. 2021. Integrating genomics and transcriptomics: Towards deciphering ADHD. *Eur Neuropsychopharmacol* 44:1-13.

Quinn, P. D., Z. Chang, K. Hur, R. D. Gibbons, B. B. Lahey, M. E. Rickert, A. Sjölander, P. Lichtenstein, H. Larsson, and B. M. D'Onofrio. 2017. ADHD medication and substance-related problems. *Am J Psychiatry* 174(9):877-885.

Rabiner, D. L., A. D. Anastopoulos, E. J. Costello, R. H. Hoyle, S. E. McCabe, and H. S. Swartzwelder. 2009. Motives and perceived consequences of nonmedical ADHD medi-cation use by college students: Are students treating themselves for attention problems? *J Atten Disord* 13(3):259-270.

Rajala, A. Z., J. B. Henriques, and L. C. Populin. 2012. Dissociative effects of methylphenidate in nonhuman primates: Trade-offs between cognitive and behavioral performance. *J Cogn Neurosci* 24(6):1371-1381.

Ramos-Quiroga, J. A., V. Nasillo, F. Fernández-Aranda, and M. Casas. 2014. Addressing the lack of studies in attention-deficit/hyperactivity disorder in adults. *Expert Review of Neurotherapeutics* 14(5):553-567.

Ramos, B. P., and A. F. Arnsten. 2007. Adrenergic pharmacology and cognition: Focus on the prefrontal cortex. *Pharmacol Ther* 113(3):523-536.

Rapoport, J. L., M. S. Buchsbaum, H. Weingartner, T. P. Zahn, C. Ludlow, and E. J. Mikkelsen. 1980. Dextroamphetamine. Its cognitive and behavioral effects in normal and hyperactive boys and normal men. *Arch Gen Psychiatry* 37(8):933-943.

Rasmussen, L., H. Zoëga, J. Hallas, and A. Pottegård. 2015. Deviant patterns of methylphenidate use in adults: A Danish nationwide registry-based drug utilization study. *Pharmacoepidemiol Drug Saf* 24(11):1189-1196.

Robe, A., A. Dobrean, I. A. Cristea, C. R. Păsărelu, and E. Predescu. 2019. Attention-deficit/hyperactivity disorder and task-related heart rate variability: A systematic review and meta-analysis. *Neurosci Biobehav Rev* 99:11-22.

Rooney, M., A. Chronis-Tuscano, and Y. Yoon. 2011. Substance use in college students with ADHD. *Journal of Attention Disorders* 16(3):221-234.

Rossom, R. C., L. I. Solberg, G. Vazquez-Benitez, A. L. Crain, A. Beck, R. Whitebird, and R. E. Glasgow. 2016. The effects of patient-centered depression care on patient satisfaction and depression remission. *Family Practice* 33(6):649-655.

Russell, G., T. Ford, R. Rosenberg, and S. Kelly. 2014. The association of attention deficit hyperactivity disorder with socioeconomic disadvantage: Alternative explanations and evidence. *J Child Psychol Psychiatry* 55(5):436-445.

Safren, S. A., S. Sprich, M. J. Mimiaga, C. Surman, L. Knouse, M. Groves, and M. W. Otto. 2010. Cognitive behavioral therapy vs relaxation with educational support for medication-treated adults with ADHD and persistent symptoms: A randomized controlled trial. *JAMA* 304(8):875-880.

SAMHSA (Substance Abuse and Mental Health Services Adminstration). 2005. *Emergency department trends from the drug abuse warning network, final estimates 1995–2002.* (SMA) 03-3780 Department of Health and Human Services.

SAMHSA. 2021. *Prescription stimulant misuse and prevention among youth and young adults.* PEP21-06-01-003 National Mental Health and Substance Use Policy Laboratory. https://store.samhsa.gov/sites/default/files/pep21-06-01-003.pdf (accessed April 30, 2024).

SAMHSA. 2023. *Key substance use and mental health indicators in the United States: Results from the 2022 national survey on drug use and health.* PEP23-07-01-006. https://www.samhsa.gov/data/report/2022-nsduh-annual-national-report (accessed April 30, 2024).

Schein, J., L. A. Adler, A. Childress, P. Gagnon-Sanschagrin, M. Davidson, F. Kinkead, M. Cloutier, A. Guérin, and P. Lefebvre. 2022. Economic burden of attention-deficit/hyperactivity disorder among adults in the United States: A societal perspective. *J Manag Care Spec Pharm* 28(2):168-179.

Schmidt, M., S. A. Schmidt, J. L. Sandegaard, V. Ehrenstein, L. Pedersen, and H. T. Sørensen. 2015. The Danish national patient registry: A review of content, data quality, and research potential. *Clin Epidemiol* 7:449-490.

Scott, D. 2023. The ongoing, unnecessary Adderall shortage, explained. *Vox.* https://www.vox.com/policy/2023/4/10/23671128/adhd-medication-adderall-shortage-2023 (accessed April 30, 2024).

Sepúlveda, D. R., L. M. Thomas, S. E. McCabe, J. A. Cranford, C. J. Boyd, and C. J. Teter. 2011. Misuse of prescribed stimulant medication for ADHD and associated patterns of substance use: Preliminary analysis among college students. *J Pharm Pract* 24(6):551-560.

Shaw, P., K. Eckstrand, W. Sharp, J. Blumenthal, J. P. Lerch, D. Greenstein, L. Clasen, A. Evans, J. Giedd, and J. L. Rapoport. 2007. Attention-deficit/hyperactivity disorder is characterized by a delay in cortical maturation. *Proc Natl Acad Sci U S A* 104(49):19649-19654.

Sheehan, D. V., Y. Lecrubier, K. H. Sheehan, P. Amorim, J. Janavs, E. Weiller, T. Hergueta, R. Baker, and G. C. Dunbar. 1998. The mini-international neuropsychiatric interview (M.I.N.I.): The development and validation of a structured diagnostic psychiatric interview for DSM-IV and ICD-10. *J Clin Psychiatry* 59 Suppl 20:22-33;quiz 34-57.

Sibley, M. H., L. E. Arnold, J. M. Swanson, L. T. Hechtman, T. M. Kennedy, E. Owens, B. S. G. Molina, P. S. Jensen, S. P. Hinshaw, A. Roy, A. Chronis-Tuscano, J. H. Newcorn, and L. A. Rohde. 2022. Variable patterns of remission from ADHD in the Multimodal Treatment study of ADHD. *Am J Psychiatry* 179(2):142-151.

Sibley, M. H., L. A. Rohde, J. M. Swanson, L. T. Hechtman, B. S. G. Molina, J. T. Mitchell, L. E. Arnold, A. Caye, T. M. Kennedy, A. Roy, and A. Stehli. 2018. Late-onset ADHD reconsidered with comprehensive repeated assessments between ages 10 and 25. *Am J Psychiatry* 175(2):140-149.

Solanto, M. V., D. J. Marks, J. Wasserstein, K. Mitchell, H. Abikoff, J. M. Alvir, and M. D. Kofman. 2010. Efficacy of meta-cognitive therapy for adult ADHD. *Am J Psychiatry* 167(8):958-968.

Solberg, B. S., A. Halmoy, A. Engeland, J. Igland, J. Haavik, and K. Klungsoyr. 2018. Gender differences in psychiatric comorbidity: A population-based study of 40 000 adults with attention deficit hyperactivity disorder. *Acta Psychiatr Scand* 137(3):176-186.

Song, P., M. Zha, Q. Yang, Y. Zhang, X. Li, and I. Rudan. 2021. The prevalence of adult attention-deficit hyperactivity disorder: A global systematic review and meta-analysis. *J Glob Health* 11:04009.

Soreff, S. 2022. *Attention deficit hyperactivity disorder (ADHD) treatment & management.* https://emedicine.medscape.com/article/289350-treatment#d8?form=fpf (accessed March 24, 2024).

Spencer, R. C., and C. W. Berridge. 2019. Receptor and circuit mechanisms underlying differential procognitive actions of psychostimulants. *Neuropsychopharmacology* 44(10):1820-1827.

Spencer, R. C., R. M. Klein, and C. W. Berridge. 2012. Psychostimulants act within the prefrontal cortex to improve cognitive function. *Biol Psychiatry* 72(3):221-227.

Spencer, T., J. Biederman, T. Wilens, R. Doyle, C. Surman, J. Prince, E. Mick, M. Aleardi, K. Herzig, and S. Faraone. 2005. A large, double-blind, randomized clinical trial of methylphenidate in the treatment of adults with attention-deficit/hyperactivity disorder. *Biol Psychiatry* 57(5):456-463.

Spencer, T. J., L. A. Adler, Q. Meihua, K. E. Saylor, T. E. Brown, J. A. Holdnack, K. J. Schuh, P. T. Trzepacz, and D. K. Kelsey. 2010. Validation of the adult ADHD investigator symptom rating scale (AISRS). *J Atten Disord* 14(1):57-68.

Sprague, R. L., and E. K. Sleator. 1977. Methylphenidate in hyperkinetic children: Differences in dose effects on learning and social behavior. *Science* 198(4323):1274-1276.

Sprich, S. E., L. E. Knouse, C. Cooper-Vince, J. Burbridge, and S. A. Safren. 2012. Description and demonstration of CBT for ADHD in adults. *Cogn Behav Pract* 17(1).

Surman, C. 2021. A controlled study of solriamfetol for ADHD in adults: Massachusetts General Hospital,. Original edition, NCT04839562.

Surman, C., C. Vaudreuil, H. Boland, L. Rhodewalt, M. DiSalvo, and J. Biederman. 2021. L-threonic acid magnesium salt supplementation in ADHD: An open-label pilot study. *J Diet Suppl* 18(2):119-131.

Surman, C. B. H., D. M. Walsh, N. Horick, M. DiSalvo, C. H. Vater, and D. Kaufman. 2023. Solriamfetol for attention-deficit/hyperactivity disorder in adults: A double-blind placebo-controlled pilot study. *J Clin Psychiatry* 84(6).

Swanson, J., L. E. Arnold, H. Kraemer, L. Hechtman, B. Molina, S. Hinshaw, P. Vitiello, P. Jensen, K. Steinhoff, M. Lerner, L. Greenhill, H. Abikoff, K. Wells, J. Epstein, G. Elliott, J. Newcorn, B. Hoza, and T. Wigal. 2008. Evidence, interpretation, and qualification from multiple reports of long-term outcomes in the multimodal treatment study of children with ADHD (MTA):Part I: Executive summary. *Journal of Attention Disorders* 12(1):4-14.

Swedish National Board of Health and Welfare. 2019. *Swedish national patient register.* https://www.socialstyrelsen.se/en/statistics-and-data/registers/national-patient-register/ (accessed April 30, 2024).

Teter, C. J., C. G. DiRaimo, B. T. West, T. S. Schepis, and S. E. McCabe. 2020. Nonmedical use of prescription stimulants among U.S. high school students to help study: Results from a national survey. *J Pharm Pract* 33(1):38-47.

Thomas, M., A. Rostain, R. Corso, T. Babcock, and M. Madhoo. 2015. ADHD in the college setting: Current perceptions and future vision. *J Atten Disord* 19(8):643-654.

Verdi, G., L. L. Weyandt, and B. M. Zavras. 2016. Non-medical prescription stimulant use in graduate students: Relationship with academic self-efficacy and psychological variables. *J Atten Disord* 20(9):741-753.

Wei, Y. J., Y. Zhu, W. Liu, R. Bussing, and A. G. Winterstein. 2018. Prevalence of and factors associated with long-term concurrent use of stimulants and opioids among adults with attention-deficit/hyperactivity disorder. *JAMA Netw Open* 1(4):e181152.

Wender, P. H. 1995. *Attention-deficit hyperactivity disorder in adults, first edition*: Oxford University Press.

Winterstein, A. G., T. Gerhard, P. Kubilis, A. Saidi, S. Linden, S. Crystal, J. Zito, J. J. Shuster, and M. Olfson. 2012. Cardiovascular safety of central nervous system stimulants in children and adolescents: Population based cohort study. *BMJ* 345:e4627.

Wolkoff Wachsman, M. 2023. DEA, drug manufacturers trade blame for generic Adderall, Vyvanse shortages. *ADDitude*.

World Federation of ADHD. 2024. *Modernizing the concept of ADHD*. https://www.adhd-federation.org/ (accessed March 24, 2024).

Yeung, A., E. Ng, and E. Abi-Jaoude. 2022. Tiktok and attention-deficit/hyperactivity disorder: A cross-sectional study of social media content quality. *Can J Psychiatry* 67(12):899-906.

Young, S., N. Adamo, B. B. Ásgeirsdóttir, P. Branney, M. Beckett, W. Colley, S. Cubbin, Q. Deeley, E. Farrag, G. Gudjonsson, P. Hill, J. Hollingdale, O. Kilic, T. Lloyd, P. Mason, E. Paliokosta, S. Perecherla, J. Sedgwick, C. Skirrow, K. Tierney, K. van Rensburg, and E. Woodhouse. 2020. Females with ADHD: An expert consensus statement taking a lifespan approach providing guidance for the identification and treatment of attention-deficit/ hyperactivity disorder in girls and women. *BMC Psychiatry* 20(1):404.

Zametkin, A. J., and M. Ernst. 1999. Problems in the management of attention-deficit-hyperactivity disorder. *N Engl J Med* 340(1):40-46.

Zhang, L., L. Li, P. Andell, M. Garcia-Argibay, P. D. Quinn, B. M. D'Onofrio, I. Brikell, R. Kuja-Halkola, P. Lichtenstein, K. Johnell, H. Larsson, and Z. Chang. 2024. Attention-deficit/hyperactivity disorder medications and long-term risk of cardiovascular diseases. *JAMA Psychiatry* 81(2):178-187.

Appendix A

Workshop Agenda

ADULT ATTENTION-DEFICIT/HYPERACTIVITY DISORDER: DIAGNOSIS, TREATMENT, AND IMPLICATIONS FOR DRUG DEVELOPMENT—A WORKSHOP

Keck Center, 500 Fifth St. NW
Washington DC, 20001

DAY 1: TUESDAY, DECEMBER 12, 2023

9:00 am   WELCOME, OPENING REMARKS, AND SETTING THE STAGE

CRAIG B.H. SURMAN, *Workshop Co-chair*
Director, Clinical and Research Program in Adult ADHD
Massachusetts General Hospital
Associate Professor of Psychiatry
Harvard Medical School

9:35 am   REGULATORY OVERVIEW

MARTA SOKOLOWSKA
Deputy Center Director
Substance Use and Behavioral Health
Center for Drug Evaluation and Research
U.S. Food and Drug Administration

SESSION I—DIAGNOSIS OF ADULTS WITH ADHD

Session Objectives:
- Discuss the criteria and available tools for diagnosis of ADHD in adults (including DSM-5 criteria, assessment tools, best practices in diagnosing the condition);
- Explore gaps and barriers when it comes to appropriate diagnosis of ADHD for different adult populations; and
- Consider the long-term public health implications of under-diagnosing, differential diagnosing, and misdiagnosing ADHD in adults and considerations for different populations.

9:55 am   **Presentation**

ANN CHILDRESS
President
Center for Psychiatry and Behavioral Medicine, Inc.
President
The American Professional Society for ADHD and Related
    Disorders

10:20 am   **Panel Discussion**

Moderator: Steve Lee, University of California, Los Angeles

Clinical Diagnosis Perspective
NAPOLEON HIGGINS
President and Chief Executive Officer
Bay Pointe Behavioral Health

Clinical Screening Perspective
SARA L. WEISENBACH
Associate Professor of Psychology in Psychiatry, Harvard
    Medical School
President, American Psychological Association, Society for
    Clinical Neuropsychology (Division 40)
Chief of Neuropsychology
McLean Hospital

Lived Experience Perspective
TAMARA ROSIER
Owner, ADHD Center of West Michigan
President
ADHD Coaches Organization

Research Perspective
MARGARET SIBLEY
Professor of Psychiatry and Behavioral Sciences
University of Washington School of Medicine

Discussion Questions:
1. Why do clinicians find it challenging to diagnose ADHD in adults (e.g., co-morbidities, differential diagnosis with other conditions such as depression, anxiety, other psychiatric conditions, and/or COVID-19)?
2. What barriers do adults experience when seeking a diagnosis of ADHD, particularly those from minority and medically underserved communities?
3. How does an ADHD diagnosis, or the lack of one, impact individuals across adulthood?
4. How is ADHD diagnosed under the DSM 5 criteria?

11:20 am   **Coffee Break**

SESSION II—MEDICATION OPTIONS FOR ADULTS WITH ADHD: RISKS AND BENEFITS

Session Objectives:
- Consider what is known and unknown about the risks and benefits of ADHD medication use in adult populations;
- Consider the public health implications for potential overprescribing of Schedule II stimulants;
- Discuss the barriers (e.g., legal, regulatory, social, cultural) to access of equitable treatment for adults with ADHD; and
- Explore approaches for alternative treatment options for adults with ADHD (e.g., non-pharmacological interventions, re-tooling of existing medications, new drug development) that may reduce the risk of harm to patients, that take into account social and cultural considerations.

11:50 am   **Presentation**

DAVID W. GOODMAN
Assistant Professor of Psychiatry and Behavioral Sciences
Johns Hopkins University School of Medicine

12:10 pm   **Panel Discussion**

Moderator: James (Jimmy) Leonard, Maryland Poison Center; University of Maryland School of Pharmacy

Lived Experience Perspective
DUANE GORDON
President
Attention Deficit Disorder Association

Clinical/Pharmacology Perspective (Medication Treatments)
ANGELA MAHOME
Staff Psychiatrist
The University of Chicago

Research/Clinical Perspective (Nonmedication Treatments/CBT)
J. RUSSELL RAMSAY
Independent Practice
Former Co-Founder, Co-Director, Adult ADHD Treatment
     and Research Program
University of Pennsylvania

Regulatory Perspective
TIFFANY R. FARCHIONE
Director, Division of Psychiatry
Center for Drug Evaluation and Research, FDA

Discussion Questions:
1. What is known and unknown about the risks and benefits of medication (stimulant and non-stimulant) use for the treatment of ADHD in adult populations?
2. What are the primary barriers (e.g., legal, regulatory, social, cultural) to appropriate treatment for adults with ADHD and how have these barriers been overcome? What are the health equity implications of these approaches?
3. How can prescribers, clinicians, and other providers be better informed regarding the treatment options available to their patients?

1:10 pm   **Lunch Break**

SESSION III—IMPLICATIONS FOR DRUG DEVELOPMENT

Session Objectives:
- Consider areas of unmet treatment needs for adults with ADHD that could potentially be addressed through new and/or improved therapeutics; and
- Explore challenges and opportunities for the development of new and improved therapeutics for the treatment of ADHD, including options that may reduce the risk of diversion.

2:00 pm   **Presentation**

CRAIG BERRIDGE
The Patricia Goldman-Rakic Professor of Psychology
University of Wisconsin, Madison

2:20 pm   **Panel Discussion**

Moderator: Stevin Zorn, MindImmune Therapeutics, Inc.

Industry Perspective
JONATHAN RUBIN
Chief Medical Officer and Senior Vice President of Research
    & Development
Supernus Pharmaceuticals

Neurobiology/Pharmacology Perspective
AMY ARNSTEN
Albert E. Kent Professor of Neuroscience and Professor of
    Psychology
Yale School of Medicine

Regulatory Perspective
ERIKA LIETZAN
William H. Pittman Professor of Law & Timothy J. Heinsz
    Professor of Law
University of Missouri School of Law

Discussion Questions:
1. How do available therapeutic treatment options meet the needs of adults with ADHD? What are the gaps/unmet medical needs?

2. How might alternative treatment options for adults with ADHD reduce the risk of harms, such as misuse potential, overdose, and toxicity?
3. What are the barriers and opportunities to the development of new medications for treating adults with ADHD?

3:20 pm   **Coffee Break**

SESSION IV—DAY 1 SYNTHESIS AND DISCUSSION

Session Objectives:
- Discuss key themes from previous workshop sessions;
- Lay out questions to be addressed; and
- Consider next step opportunities for improving the diagnosis and treatment of adults with ADHD; implications for drug development.

3:50 pm   **Panel Discussion**

Moderator: Craig B. H. Surman, Massachusetts General Hospital; Harvard Medical School

Pharmacology Perspective
ALMUT WINTERSTEIN
Director, Center for Drug Evaluation and Safety (CoDES) and Consortium for Medical Marijuana Clinical Outcomes Research
Distinguished Professor, Pharmaceutical Outcomes and Policy
University of Florida

Industry Perspective
DAVID BAKER
Former Pharmaceutical Executive – Shire, Alcobra, Vallon Pharmaceuticals
Board Member
Edge Foundation

Lived Experience Perspective
KOFI OBENG
Executive Director
Attention Deficit Disorder Association

Resources and Education Perspective
SUNNY PATEL
Senior Advisor for Children, Youth and Families
SAMHSA

Research Perspective
MARY SOLANTO
Professor of Pediatrics and Psychiatry
Zucker School of Medicine at Hofstra-Northwell

Discussion Questions:
1. Based on the day's sessions, what are the main themes you heard regarding the diagnosis, treatment, and drug development for ADHD in adult populations? What questions remain?
2. How can the use of a health equity framework help the those with adult ADHD, health professionals, and others better understand the social, political, economic, and environmental factors impacting the diagnosis and treatment of adult ADHD?
3. How do we bridge the gap from where we are now to where we want to be? What is needed and from whom?
4. What are some key things from today's sessions we should keep in mind as we move into Day 2?

4:35 pm   **Audience Q&A**

DAY 1 CLOSING REMARKS

CARLOS BLANCO, *Workshop Co-chair*
Director, Division of Epidemiology, Services, and Prevention
    Research
National Institute on Drug Abuse, NIH

5:00 pm   **Adjourn Workshop Day 1**

5:00 pm   **Reception**

DAY 2: WEDNESDAY, DECEMBER 13, 2023

8:30 am   OPENING REMARKS

CARLOS BLANCO, *Workshop Co-chair*
Director, Division of Epidemiology, Services, and Prevention
    Research
National Institute on Drug Abuse, NIH

8:40 am   FIRESIDE CHAT

CARLOS BLANCO, *Workshop Co-chair*
Director, Division of Epidemiology, Services, and Prevention
    Research
National Institute on Drug Abuse, NIH

EVELYN POLK GREEN
Immediate Past President;
Attention Deficit Disorder Association
Past President;
Children & Adults with Attention Deficit/Hyperactivity
    Disorder

SESSION V—ENABLING ACCESS TO RESOURCES AND SHARED DECISION MAKING FOR ADULTS WITH ADHD AND THEIR PROVIDERS

Session Objective:
- Share perspectives and available resources for prescribers, clinicians, and patients on the risks and benefits of ADHD medication use in adults, particularly for underserved populations;
- Discuss practical approaches that have helped overcome barriers (e.g., stigma, misdiagnosis) to appropriate diagnosis and treatment of adults with ADHD; and
- Consider opportunities to enable shared decision making between patients and their providers regarding the diagnosis and treatment of ADHD.

9:20 am   **Presentation**

MARK OLFSON
Professor of Psychiatry, Medicine, and Law;
Professor of Epidemiology
Columbia University

9:40 am   **Presentation**

LARA ROBINSON
Behavioral Scientist
National Center on Birth Defects and Developmental
    Disabilities, CDC

9:55 am   **Panel Discussion**

*Moderator: Andrea Chronis-Tuscano, University of Maryland,
Department of Psychology*

Lived Experience Perspective
KYLIE BARRON

Clinical Perspective
BRANDI WALKER
Chief Executive Officer
Marie Pauline Consulting, LLC

Psychiatrist Perspective
BENJAMIN CHEYETTE
Psychiatrist
Director of ADHD Programming
Mindful Health Solutions

Telehealth and Social Media Perspective
JESSICA GOLD
Associate Professor, Department of Psychiatry, University of
    Tennessee Health and Science Center
Chief Wellness Officer
University of Tennessee (UT) System
(*As of* 2/1/2024)

Discussion Questions:
1. What methods and/or systems are in place to support
   prescribers, clinicians, and other providers who diagnose
   and treat adults with ADHD? What else is needed?
2. Are there lessons learned from the diagnosis and treatment
   of pediatric populations that may be applicable for adult
   populations?

3. What approaches have and/or could help support adults with ADHD make informed decisions about the risks and benefits of ADHD medication use?
4. How can we best disseminate evidence-based educational materials/content about adult ADHD to patients (including those from diverse backgrounds) so that they can engage in informed discussions around their care?

SESSION VI—PUBLIC HEALTH CONSIDERATIONS AND HARM REDUCTION STRATEGIES FOR ADHD MEDICATION USE

Session Objectives:
- Share perspectives on the causes, perceptions, consequences, and health equity implications of non-medical use of prescription stimulants;
- Discuss what is known and unknown about the intersection of ADHD medication use (medical and non-medical) and opioid use; and
- Consider how strategies to reduce the misuse of ADHD medications could impact public health (e.g., limiting patient access to medication, exacerbating existing health inequities).

10:55 am   **Presentation**

BROOKE MOLINA
Professor of Psychiatry, Psychology, Pediatrics, Clinical & Translational Science
University of Pittsburgh

11:15 am   **Panel Discussion**

Moderator: Taleed El-Sabawi, Florida International University

Clinical Perspective
ROBIN WEISS
Private Practice of Psychiatry
Past President
Maryland Psychiatric Society

Lived Experience Perspective
PATRICK KELLY

Research/Community Health Perspective
RYAN MCNEIL
Associate Professor, Director of Harm Reduction Research
Yale School of Medicine

Research/Clinical Perspective
KEVIN ANTSHEL
Professor of Psychology and Associate Department Chair
Syracuse University

Discussion Questions:
1. What is known and unknown about the intersection of ADHD medication use (medical and non-medical) and opioid use?
2. What are public health and health equity implications of not appropriately treating adults with ADHD?
3. What strategies (e.g., public health efforts, regulatory policies) have been deployed to reduce the misuse of ADHD medications and what was the impact on people with ADHD? What was the impact on public health?

12:15 pm   **Coffee Break**

SESSION VII—DAY 2 SYNTHESIS AND DISCUSSION

Session Objectives:
- Discuss key themes from previous workshop sessions; and
- Consider next step opportunities for improving the diagnosis and treatment of adults with ADHD.

12:45 pm   **Panel Discussion**

Moderator: Carlos Blanco, National Institute on Drug Abuse, NIH

Clinical Perspective—ADHD in underserved populations
JOSEPH SCHATZ
Director, Psychiatric/Mental Health Nurse Practitioner Track
University of Pennsylvania School of Nursing

Lived Experience Perspective
TALEED EL-SABAWI
Assistant Professor of Law
Florida International University

Pharmacology Perspective
MATTHEW RUDORFER
Chief, Psychopharmacology, Somatic, and Integrated
    Treatment Research Program
National Institute of Mental Health, NIH

Research Perspective
AMELIA ARRIA
Director, Center on Young Adult Health and Development
Professor, Department of Behavioral and Community Health
University of Maryland School of Public Health

Family Medicine Perspective
LATASHA SELIBY PERKINS
Assistant Professor of Medicine
Georgetown University School of Medicine

Discussion Questions:
1. Based on the day's sessions, what are the main themes you heard regarding enabling access to resources, shared decision making, and strategies to reduce the misuse of ADHD medications for adults with ADHD? What questions remain?
2. How can the use of a health equity framework help those with adult ADHD, health professionals, and others better understand the social, political, economic, and environmental factors impacting the health and overall well-being of adults with ADHD?
3. Considering everything you've heard over the past day and a half, what is important for the FDA to know as it relates to diagnosis, treatment, and drug development for adult ADHD?

1:35 pm   **Audience Q&A**

1:50 pm   CLOSING REMARKS

MARTA SOKOLOWSKA
Deputy Center Director
Substance Use and Behavioral Health
Center for Drug Evaluation and Research
U.S. Food and Drug Administration

CRAIG B.H. SURMAN, *Workshop Co-chair*
Director, Clinical and Research Program in Adult ADHD
Massachusetts General Hospital
Associate Professor of Psychiatry
Harvard Medical School

2:00 pm   **Adjourn Day 2**

Appendix B

Biographical Sketches of the Workshop Planning Committee, Speakers, Panelists, and Staff

PLANNING COMMITTEE BIOSKETCHES

CARLOS BLANCO, M.D., PH.D., (*Co-Chair*) is the Director of the Division of Epidemiology, Services, and Prevention Research at the National Institute on Drug Abuse (NIDA), a component of the National Institutes of Health (NIH). Blanco is a national known expert in the epidemiology and treatment of addictive disorders with and without comorbid disorders. His accomplishments include, among others, a detailed examination of the course and stages of substance use disorders, the development of methods to quantify the generalizability of clinical trials, the development and testing of interventions that combine motivational interviewing with cognitive-behavioral therapy to improve retention and outcome in individuals with addictive disorders, and the creation of a virtual map of psychiatric disorders, based on empirical data, to guide research into the causes of mental disorders. Prior to joining NIDA, Blanco was professor of psychiatry at Columbia University Medical Center and a Research Psychiatrist at the New York State Psychiatric Institute. He is a graduate of Universidad Autónoma de Madrid (Spain) and completed his psychiatry residency at Columbia University, where he also completed a research fellowship. Blanco has authored more than 200 peer-reviewed publications.

CRAIG B. H. SURMAN, M.D., (*Co-Chair*) is Director of the Clinical and Research Program in Adult ADHD and Staff Neuropsychiatrist at Massachusetts General Hospital. Surman investigates and educates disorders of self-regulation as an associate professor of psychiatry at Harvard

Medical School. He is co-chair of the Children and Adults with ADHD (CHADD) Professional Advisory Board, and a former board member for the American Professional Society of ADHD and Related Disorders (APSARD), where he serves on the Board nominating committee. With international experts, he created "ADHD in Adults: A Practical Guide to Evaluation and Management." An advocate for evidence-informed care, he co-authored "FAST MINDS: How to Thrive If You Have ADHD (or Think You Might)." Contributing to more than 50 investigations, he has illuminated the connection between Adult ADHD and comorbidities, and clarified the promise of novel behavioral, pharmacologic, and nutraceutical interventions for ADHD. Surman recently piloted application of remote digital measurement in ADHD treatment monitoring and in a clinical trial. To understand factors contributing to national ADHD treatment trends, he is currently collaborating with the Centers for Disease Control. He is a graduate of Oberlin College, University of Massachusetts Medical School, and completed residency and fellowship training at Harvard Medical School.

AMY F. T. ARNSTEN, PH.D., is the Albert E. Kent Professor of Neuroscience at the Yale University School of Medicine. She is an international expert on the molecular regulation of the primate prefrontal cortex, the brain region most often afflicted in ADHD, and has developed a nonstimulant treatment for ADHD, guanfacine (Intuniv), that was FDA-approved for this indication in 2009. This is one of the few examples where knowledge arising from basic science has successfully translated to a treatment for human cognitive disorders. Guanfacine is also being used off-label to treat other prefrontal cortical disorders, including cognitive deficits from long COVID. Arnsten is a member of the National Academy of Medicine and the recipient of the Goldman-Rakic Prize for Outstanding Research in Cognitive Neuroscience. She received her B.A. in neuroscience from Brown University in 1976, creating the neuroscience major, and her Ph.D. in neuroscience from University of California, San Diego, in 1982.

ANDREA M. CHRONIS-TUSCANO, PH.D., is the Joel and Kim Feller Professor of Psychology at the University of Maryland (UMD), College Park, and the Director of the UMD Students Understanding College Choices Encouraging and Executing Decisions for Success (SUCCEEDS) College Attention-Deficit/ Hyperactivity Disorder (ADHD) Clinic. Chronis-Tuscano's research focuses broadly on understanding early predictors of developmental outcomes for children with ADHD (including depression and alcohol/substance use) and developing novel treatments which target these early risk and protective factors. Much of this research has addressed issues related to maternal parenting and psychopathology (namely, maternal depression and ADHD).

Most recently, she has utilized hybrid effectiveness-implementation designs to develop treatments that can be implemented in community settings such as pediatrics and schools. Chronis-Tuscano is also the president-elect of the Society for Clinical Child and Adolescent Psychology (APA Division 53); Past-president of the International Society for Research in Child and Adolescent Psychopathology; past associate editor of the *Journal of Consulting & Clinical Psychology*; fellow of the Association for Psychological Science; fellow of the Association for Behavioral & Cognitive Therapies (ABCT); former associate editor of the *Journal of Clinical Child & Adolescent Psychology*; and former standing member of the National Institute of Mental Health (NIMH) Mental Health Services Research (SERV) review committee. She is the recipient of multiple National Institute of Health (NIH) grants and has served on several NIH review committees relevant to developmental psychopathology and interventions.

TALEED EL-SABAWI, J.D., PH.D., is an interdisciplinary scholar with degrees in public health, health services management and policy and a doctoral cognate in political science. Her area of expertise is in addiction and mental health policy, politics, and law, specifically contemporary issues at the intersection of addiction, race, and policing. El-Sabawi, a person with lived experience with ADD and adult diagnosis of ADD, has been personally affected by the stimulant shortage. In addition to her scholarship, El-Sabawi has advised federal, state, and local governments, including the Office of National Drug Control Policy, U.S. Department of Justice, Jails Division, and North Carolina's Attorney General's Office. She has drafted a model law for the creation of non-police behavioral health crisis response teams, which is being circulated by organizers in New Orleans (LA), Nashville (TN), Columbus (OH), Chicago (IL), Boston (MA), and Durham (NC). El-Sabawi is on the advisory circle of the North Carolina Urban Survivors Union, a chapter of the Urban Survivors Union, serves on the Board of Directors for Next Distro, and frequently works alongside persons who use drugs advocating for policy reform.

EVELYN POLK GREEN, M.S.ED., is a past national president of both the Attention Deficit Disorder Association (ADDA) and Children and Adults with Attention-Deficit/Hyperactivity Disorder (CHADD). She is an adult with attention-deficit/hyperactivity disorder (ADHD), and the mother of two adult sons both of whom also have ADHD. Active in ADHD and mental health advocacy for close to 30 years, she has served as a leader representing the family voice in the ADHD and mental health communities in many capacities, including as a member of the Network on Children's Mental Health Services funded by the MacArthur Foundation. She frequently represents the family/consumer perspective on mental health issues and often speaks to audiences and the media on a variety of topics. She has been focused on the challenges of ADHD in minority, poor, and other underserved populations throughout her advocacy career. She is the recipient of several honors for her volunteer work in mental health and education, including the Beacon College Achieving Lifetime Vision and Excellence (ALiVE) Award for her advocacy work on behalf of children and adults with learning differences and ADHD. Green works as an administrator with the Chicago Public Schools, planning professional development programs for early childhood special education professionals and families. She holds bachelor and master's degrees from National Louis University and a master's degree from Northern Illinois University.

STEVE S. LEE, PH.D., is a professor of psychology and the director of clinical psychology training in the Department of Psychology at the University of California, Los Angeles (UCLA). He completed his undergraduate degree in psychology at the University of Chicago, his doctoral training in clinical psychology at the University of California, Berkeley, and then post-doctoral training in psychiatric genetics at the University of Chicago. He is an expert in the origins, development, and outcomes of youth with ADHD and related disruptive behavior and emotional problems. His program of research leverages diverse methods spanning microanalytic coding of behavior and longitudinal designs to meta-analytic reviews. Lee was past secretary/treasurer of the International Society for Research in Child and Adolescent Psychopathology and past-president of the Society for Clinical Child and Adolescent Psychology. He was the recipient of the 2021 Mavis Hetherington Award for Excellence in Applied Developmental Science from the American Psychological Association.

JAMES (JIMMY) LEONARD, PHARM.D., DABAT, is the Director of Clinical Services for the Maryland Poison Center and an associate professor at the University of Maryland School of Pharmacy. His practice and research focus on management and prevention of poisoning including exploratory ingestions in children, medication errors in all populations, and self-harm attempts in adolescents and adults. He is a member of the American Association of Clinical Toxicology and America's Poison Centers (formerly American Association of Poison Control Centers). He is the chair of the data access committee for America's Poison Centers. He attended Washington State University for undergraduate and pharmacy school, followed by a one-year hospital residency in Olympia, Washington. After completion of residency, he did a two-year fellowship in Clinical Toxicology from 2017 to 2019 before joining the staff at the Maryland Poison Center and subsequently the faculty at the University of Maryland School of Pharmacy.

TAMARA ROSIER, PH.D., is founder of the Attention-Deficit/Hyperactivity Disorder (ADHD) Center of West Michigan, where she and her staff of coaches and therapists work with individuals with ADHD (and their families) to learn strategies and develop new skills to live effectively with ADHD. Rosier's experiences as a college administrator, a professor, and a high school teacher afforded her valuable insight into ADHD and how it affects one's life. She is also the president of the ADHD Coaches Organization and co-chair of the International Conference on ADHD. She has published numerous articles about living with ADHD and frequently speaks at conferences. Her book, *Your Brain's Not Broken*, provides strategies for managing the emotional aspects of ADHD.

MATTHEW RUDORFER, M.D., is a longtime Medical Officer at the National Institute of Mental Health (NIMH), and serves as Chief of the Psychopharmacology, Somatic, and Integrated Treatment Research Program, Treatment and Preventive Interventions Research Branch, in the NIMH Division of Services and Intervention Research. In this capacity he oversees grants and contracts supporting clinical trials, including pharmacotherapy studies, primarily in adults suffering from a range of mental disorders. In the past he served for a dozen years as Program Chair or Co-Chair of the annual New Clinical Drug Evaluation Unit (NCDEU) national treatment research meeting, which brought together clinical investigators from Government, academia, and industry. Following a term as Member and Chair of the FDA Psychiatric Drugs Advisory Committee, he remains an ad hoc voting member, providing uncompensated service to multiple advisory committees over the years. He is also past Editor-in-Chief of the peer-reviewed Psychopharmacology Bulletin. At present, he serves on the editorial boards of CNS Drugs and the Journal of ECT. In addition to his work at NIMH, Dr. Rudorfer maintains a small private practice in psychiatry and psychopharmacology. He is Board-Certified in Psychiatry and Clinical Pharmacology and is a member of the American Society of Clinical Pharmacology and Therapeutics (ASCPT), the American Society of Clinical Psychopharmacology (ASCP), the Society of Biological Psychiatry, and the American Psychiatric Association. At present, he is Chair of the Continuing Medical Education (CME) Committee of the Washington Psychiatric Society. After receiving his medical degree from the State University of New York, Downstate College of Medicine, Rudorfer undertook his residency in Psychiatry at Washington University in St. Louis, followed by a National Institute of General Medical Science (NIGMS) Fellowship in Clinical Pharmacology, prior to launching his research career, studying novel medications for the treatment of mood disorders, in the NIMH intramural program.

ALMUT G. WINTERSTEIN, PH.D., is distinguished professor in pharmaceutical outcomes and policy, affiliate professor in Epidemiology, and the founding director of the Center for Drug Evaluation and Safety at the University of Florida. In 2017, she was named the Dr. Robert and Barbara Crisafi Chair for Medication Safety in recognition of her research on drug safety and on devising ways to improve medication use. Winterstein's research interests center on the post-marketing evaluation of drugs in pediatrics and pregnancy, infectious disease and psychiatry and the evaluation of policy surrounding medication use using real-world data. As expert in drug safety, she has chaired the Food and Drug Administration's Drug Safety and Risk Management Advisory Committee from 2012–2018. Winterstein was inducted as a fellow of the International Society of Pharmacoepidemiology in 2013 and served as president of the society from 2019–2020. Since 2019 she serves as director of the Consortium for Medical Marijuana Clinical Outcomes Research, a state-funded consortium of 9 universities in Florida. In 2022 she was inducted in the Academy of Science, Engineering and Medicine in Florida. She received her pharmacy degree from Friedrich Wilhelm University in Bonn, Germany, and her Ph.D. in pharmacoepidemiology from Humboldt University in Berlin.

STEVIN H. ZORN, PH.D., is currently president and CEO of MindImmune Therapeutics. Zorn is a neuropharmacologist with extensive executive experience throughout the pharmaceutical value chain and has more than 30 years of drug discovery and drug development success across a broad range of neuro and psychiatric disorders. Prior to co-founding MindImmune Therapeutics in 2016, Zorn was Executive Vice President and Site head for Neuroscience Research for Lundbeck's USA Research Site, Lundbeck Research U.S.A., and board member for Lundbeck USA. He has been a member of Lundbeck's Global Research Committee, Development Committee, Research and Development (R&D) Management Group, the R&D Executive Committee and U.S. R&D Management Group. He conceived of and built one of the first Neuroinflammation Disease Biology Units in the industry. There he established a talented group of scientists that brought together disciplines of immunology, inflammation, and neuroscience to capitalize on the recently growing knowledge base showing the relationship between neuroinflammation and central nervous system diseases to advance new approaches for the treatment of mental illness. This became Lundbeck U.S.A.'s primary area of focus. Prior to Lundbeck, Zorn was with Pfizer Global Research and Development for nearly 20 years. He held positions including head of General Pharmacology, Alzheimer's Disease Clinical Development Team Leader, Head of Psychotherapeutics Biology, Head of Neuroscience Therapeutics, Co-Chair of the Global Neuroscience Therapeutic Area Leadership Team including accountability for all R&D

as well as commercialization, and was Vice President and Global Therapeutic Area Head for Central Nervous System Disorders Research at Pfizer including chair of the Global Research Therapeutic Area Leadership Team. Zorn became Pfizer's first global head of Neuroscience Research, was co-architect of what became the company's overall Neuroscience area strategy and co-led the second largest and among the most productive therapeutic areas at Pfizer. As member of the Discovery Research Management Team of the Ann Arbor Pfizer site, Zorn was also jointly accountable for site deliverables from five therapeutic areas: neuroscience, cardiovascular, inflammation, dermatology, and infectious diseases. Across his industry career, Zorn shepherded or led research generating dozens of drug candidates from Lundbeck and Pfizer in clinical development for multiple indications; many have progressed to phase II/III or have advanced into commercialization. In conjunction with his responsibilities as President and CEO of MindImmune Therapeutics, Inc., Zorn is a Ryan Research Professor of Neuroscience at the University of Rhode Island. Zorn received a B.S. degree in chemistry from Lafayette College, Easton, Pennsylvania, and M.S. and Ph.D. degrees in neurotoxicology and neuropharmacology, respectively, from the University of Texas Graduate School of Biomedical Sciences, Houston, Texas. Subsequent postdoctoral research studies centered on basic research of brain and intracellular neuronal signaling mechanisms at the Rockefeller University, New York, New York, in the laboratory of Paul Greengard (Nobel Laureate).

SPEAKER AND PANELIST BIOSKETCHES

KEVIN ANTSHEL, PH.D., is a professor of psychology and associate department chair at Syracuse University. Antshel's programmatic line of research focuses on better understanding the heterogeneity of ADHD with a specific emphasis on college student attention-deficit/hyperactivity disorder (ADHD). He is a board-certified clinical child and adolescent psychologist who maintains an active clinical practice devoted to ADHD.

AMELIA M. ARRIA, PH.D., is a professor and the director of the Center on Young Adult Health and Development in the Department of Behavioral and Community Health at the University of Maryland School of Public Health. Her research focuses on mental health and substance use problems among adolescents and young adults, including the nonmedical use of prescription drugs. Her most recent work has clarified the impact of substance use on academic achievement. She led the NIDA-funded prospective College Life Study, which investigated the behavioral health of 1,253 college students through their young adult years. She is the co-leader of the Maryland Collaborative, a network of 19 colleges working to promote college student health with science-based strategies. She has authored more than 185 peer-reviewed publications. Her work has relevance to parents, communities, educational professionals, and policymakers. She received a B.S. from Cornell University, a PhD in epidemiology from the University of Pittsburgh and postdoctoral training in psychiatric epidemiology at Johns Hopkins University.

DAVID BAKER, MBA, has more than 30 years of executive, operational and commercial leadership experience in the biopharmaceutical industry. He has been directly involved with the development and commercialization of multiple attention-deficit/hyperactivity disorder (ADHD) medications, including Adderall XR® and Vyvanse®, the two most successful ADHD brands based on annual revenue. He currently serves as an advisor to start-up life sciences companies, as a board director, and as an angel investor. Previously, he was the co-founder and CEO of Vallon Pharmaceuticals, which worked to develop abuse-deterrent stimulants for ADHD. Prior to that, he was Chief Commercial Officer and interim CEO of Alcobra Ltd., a pharmaceutical company developing a novel non-stimulant for ADHD. He worked at Shire Plc for 10 years as Vice President of Commercial Strategy and New Business in the Neuroscience Business Unit, Global General Manager for Vyvanse® and Vice President, ADHD Marketing. Prior to Shire, he worked at Merck & Co. in marketing, sales, market research, and business development. Mr. Baker earned a BA in economics and computer science from Duke University, and an MBA from Duke's Fuqua School of Business.

KYLIE BARRON, M.P.H., was diagnosed with attention-deficit/hyperactivity disorder (ADHD) as a teenager and feels most at home working within the ADHD community. She is the Vice President of the Attention Deficit Disorder Association (ADDA) and has served as the Marketing Communications Chair on the Board of Directors since 2018. As a public health marketing professional, Kylie's work combines innovative marketing strategies with forward-thinking health promotion techniques to catalyze positive health behavior changes within hard-to-reach audiences. Kylie spends her off-time contributing to her family's business and working as an Advanced EMT in her community.

CRAIG BERRIDGE, PH.D., is the Patricia Goldman-Rakic Professor of Psychology at the University of Wisconsin-Madison. He has long-standing expertise in the behavioral and physiological actions of central catecholamines and catecholamine-targeting drugs, particularly psychostimulants. His lab was at the forefront in the development of experimental approaches for studying the neural mechanisms that support the procognitive actions of psychostimulants used in the treatment of attention-deficit/hyperactivity disorder (ADHD). This research definitively demonstrates that psychostimulants act directly in the prefrontal cortex to promote higher cognitive processes and identifies the catecholamine receptor mechanisms that underlie these actions. More recently he has used this information to identify non-catecholamine neurotransmitters within the prefrontal cortex that regulate higher cognitive function and that could be targeted in the development of novel treatments for cognitive dysfunction associated with ADHD.

ROBERT CALIFF, M.D., MACC, NAM, is Commissioner of Food and Drugs. President Joe Biden nominated Califf to head the U.S. Food and Drug Administration and Califf was sworn in on February 17, 2022. Previously, he served as Commissioner of Food and Drugs from February 2016 to January 2017. As the top official of the FDA, Califf is committed to strengthening programs and policies that enable the agency to carry out its mission to protect and promote the public health. Califf served as the FDA's Deputy Commissioner for Medical Products and Tobacco from February 2015 until his first appointment as Commissioner in February 2016. Prior to rejoining the FDA, Califf was head of medical strategy and Senior Advisor at Alphabet Inc., contributing to strategy and policy for its health subsidiaries Verily Life Sciences and Google Health. He joined Alphabet in 2019, after serving as a professor of medicine and vice chancellor for clinical and translational research at Duke University. He also served as director of the Duke Translational Medicine Institute and founding director of the Duke Clinical Research Institute. A nationally and internationally recognized expert in cardiovascular medicine, health outcomes research, health care quality, and clinical research, Califf has led many landmark clinical trials and is one of the most frequently cited authors in biomedical science, with more than 1,300 publications in the peer-reviewed literature. Califf became a Member of the National Academy of Medicine (formerly known as the Institute of Medicine [IOM]) in 2016, one of the highest honors in the fields of health and medicine. Califf has served on numerous IOM committees, and he has served as a member of the FDA Cardiorenal Advisory Panel and the FDA Science Board's Subcommittee on Science and Technology. He has also served on the Board of Scientific Counselors for the National Library of Medicine, as well as on advisory committees for the National Cancer Institute, the National Heart, Lung, and Blood Institute, the National Institute of Environmental Health Sciences and the Council of the National Institute on Aging. While at Duke, Califf led major initiatives aimed at improving methods and infrastructure for clinical research, including the Clinical Trials Transformation Initiative (CTTI), a public–private partnership co-founded by the

FDA and Duke. He also served as the principal investigator for Duke's Clinical and Translational Science Award and the NIH Health Care Systems Research Collaboratory Coordinating Center. Califf is a graduate of Duke University School of Medicine. He completed a residency in internal medicine at the University of California, San Francisco, and a fellowship in cardiology at Duke.

BENJAMIN CHEYETTE, M.D., PH.D., spent approximately 20 years as faculty in the UCSF Department of Psychiatry, both as an Attending and as an NIH-funded Independent Investigator focused on genetically engineered mouse models of neurodevelopment. He retired as Professor Emeritus in 2018 and has since worked in the non-profit and private sectors treating insured psychiatric outpatients. Since Jan 2021 he has been the attention-deficit/hyperactivity disorder (ADHD) Program Director at Mindful Health Solutions (MHS), an interventional (TMS & esketamine) psychiatry practice with approximately 100 providers in 4 states. At MHS he has developed training for adult psychiatrists and PMHNPs who typically arrive unprepared to diagnose and treat adult ADHD—the primary diagnosis in >15% of MHS patients and a highly comorbid secondary diagnosis in patients presenting with depression or anxiety—in line with recent US epidemiological data. MHS emphasizes Measurement-Based Care; Dr. Cheyette has accordingly developed a rapid self-administered ADHD symptom-tracking scale (the HII-5) closely modeled on the widely used PHQ-9 for depression and GAD-7 for anxiety.

ANN CHILDRESS, M.D., is President of the American Professional Society of Attention-Deficit/Hyperactivity Disorder (ADHD) and Related Disorders and is in private practice in Las Vegas, Nevada, where she specializes in the treatment of attention-deficit/hyperactivity disorder (ADHD). She has adjunct faculty appointments at the Kirk Kerkorian School of Medicine at UNLV and Touro University Nevada College of Osteopathic Medicine. Childress is board certified in psychiatry, with a subspecialty in child and adolescent psychiatry. She has authored more than 100 publications on the topic of ADHD. As an investigator, she has participated in approximately 250 clinical trials.

TIFFANY R. FARCHIONE, M.D., received her medical degree from Wayne State University in Detroit, Michigan, and completed adult residency and child and adolescent fellowship training at the University of Pittsburgh's Western Psychiatric Institute and Clinic (now UPMC Western Psychiatric Hospital). Farchione is board certified in both general and child & adolescent psychiatry. Prior to joining FDA in 2010, she was affiliated with the University of Pittsburgh Medical Center and was on the faculty of the University of Pittsburgh. As the Director of the Division of Psychiatry in the Office of Neuroscience at FDA, Farchione is involved in the oversight of new drug review for all psychiatric drug development activities conducted under investigational new drug applications (INDs), and the review of all new drug application (NDAs) and supplements for new psychiatric drug claims.

JESSICA GOLD, M.D., M.S., will be the Chief Wellness Officer of the University of Tennessee System and an associate professor in the Department of Psychiatry at the University of Tennessee Health and Science Center as of February 1, 2024. She was previously the Director of Wellness, Engagement, and Outreach at Washington University in St. Louis School of Medicine. She works clinically as an outpatient psychiatrist and sees faculty, staff, hospital employees, and their dependents, with special emphasis on college-aged kids. She also writes and is a regular expert for the media on mental health and been featured in, among others, *The New York Times, The Atlantic, NPR, PBS News Hour, The Washington Post,* and *SELF*. Gold is a graduate of the University of Pennsylvania with a B.A. and M.S in anthropology, the Yale School of Medicine, and completed her residency training in adult psychiatry at Stanford University where she served as chief resident.

DAVID W. GOODMAN, M.D., is assistant professor of psychiatry and behavioral sciences at the Johns Hopkins University School of Medicine and clinical associate professor of psychiatry and behavioral sciences at the Norton School of Medicine, State University of New York–Upstate. An internationally recognized expert, he has presented more than 600 lectures to medical specialists, authored peer-reviewed scientific papers, conducted clinical research on several of the ADHD medications now on the market, serves as a consultant to the NFL, widely quoted in national media, teaches fourth-year psychiatric residents at the Johns Hopkins School of Medicine and State University of New York-Upstate, serves as the Treasurer of APSARD (American Professional Society for ADHD and Related Disorders), and a member of the APSARD Task Force for the development of the APSARD's U.S. Clinical Practice Guidelines for the Diagnosis and Treatment of ADHD in adults.

DUANE GORDON is President of the Attention Deficit Disorder Association (ADDA). An adult with attention-deficit/hyperactivity disorder (ADHD) himself, he has 25 years' experience as an advocate for adults with ADHD. He was a founding member and co-leader of the Montreal Adult ADHD Support Group from 1998 to 2020. He joined ADDA in 2004 and began volunteering with ADDA in 2005. He joined ADDA's

Communication team, volunteering as a writer, and later taking on the role of newsletter editor. In 2011, he joined ADDA's Board as Chair of Communication. The ADDA Board of Directors is a team of exceptional leaders with ADHD, and Duane is proud and grateful they chose him to lead as president in 2016. Gordon is an in-demand speaker on topics related to adult ADHD. He retired early from a career as a technology consultant to pursue his passions as an ADHD advocate and artist. He lives in Montreal, Canada.

NAPOLEON HIGGINS, M.D., is a child, adolescent and adult psychiatrist in Houston, Texas. He is the owner of Bay Pointe Behavioral Health Services and South East Houston Research Group. Higgins received his M.D. from Meharry Medical College in Nashville, Tennessee, and he completed his residency in adult psychiatry and his fellowship in child and adolescent psychiatry at University of Texas Medical Branch at Galveston. He is the Executive Director of the Black Psychiatrists of America, CEO of Global Health Psychiatry, President of the Black Psychiatrists of Greater Houston, and Past President of the Caucus of Black Psychiatrists of the American Psychiatric Association. Dr. Higgins is co-author of *Bree's Journey to Joy: A Story about Childhood Grief and Depression, How Amari Learned to Love School Again: A Story about ADHD, Mind Matters: A Resource Guide to Psychiatry for Black Communities* and author of *Transition 2 Practice: 21 Things Every Doctor Must Know In Contract Negotiations and the Job Search*. He also specializes in nutrition and health to improve patients' lives mentally and physically. He emphasizes that good mental and physical health are key in the practice of psychiatry and medicine. Higgins has worked with and founded many programs that help to direct inner-city young men and women to aspire to go to college and finish their educational goals. He has worked with countless community mentoring programs and has special interest in trauma, racism, and inner-city issues and how they affect minority and disadvantaged children and communities.

PATRICK KELLY is a patient advocate who was diagnosed with attention-deficit/hyperactivity disorder (ADHD) in first grade. He started simulant therapy at diagnosis, which he continues to this day. He began to take an active role in his ADHD management seven years ago while he was getting sober. These two things had a synergistic effect; a 12-step program helped with ADHD management, and ADHD management helped sobriety. He first became involved in the Attention Deficit Disorder Association (ADDA) in 2020 and has served as a facilitator for the Young People's Peer Support group since 2022. Despite major challenges due to ADHD and addiction, Kelly is a college graduate who lived overseas for a year and maintains close friendships. He enjoys kayaking, self-improvement, and staying up-to-date on current events and ADHD research.

ERIKA LIETZAN, J.D., M.A., is the William H. Pittman Professor of Law and Timothy J. Heinsz Professor of Law at the University of Missouri School of Law. She focuses her scholarship and teaching primarily in the areas of health law and policy, with a special focus on FDA regulation, administrative law, and intellectual property. She has published extensively on federal regulation of biopharmaceutical research, development, and approval, as well as innovation policy. Before joining academia, she practiced law for eighteen years, including eight years as a partner in the food and drug group at Covington & Burling. She has been consistently identified by her peers in private practice as a "Best Lawyer in America" in the categories of FDA law (since 2013) and Biotechnology Law (since 2007).

ANGELA MAHOME, M.D., is the is board-certified in General Psychiatry and Child and Adolescent Psychiatry. Currently, she works in Student Wellness at the University of Chicago and as a consultant for Danville School District 118 in downstate Illinois. Upon graduating from the Medical College of Georgia, she completed her residency and fellowship at the University of Chicago Hospitals. While providing outpatient care, she received numerous invitations from schools to speak to educators about attention-deficit/hyperactivity disorder (ADHD) and while working as the medical director for an inpatient Adolescent Behavioral Health Unit, she gave a presentation to the 256 Chicago Public School nurses on ADHD which was well received. Mahome has previously served on the ADHD Expert Speaker's Bureau for two major pharmaceutical companies and is currently on the ADDA (Attention Deficit Disorder Association) medical advisory board. She is a member of the American Academy of Child and Adolescent Psychiatry.

RYAN MCNEIL, PH.D., is an associate professor of internal medicine, public health, and anthropology at Yale University. Through his community-engaged qualitative and ethnographic research, he examines social, structural, and environmental influences on drug-related harms and the implementation of substance use interventions. His recent work has examined dynamics shaping stimulant- and polysubstance use–related harms, as well as the potential uses of prescription stimulants for addressing stimulant-related harms.

BROOKE MOLINA, PH.D., is professor of psychiatry, psychology, and pediatrics at the University of Pittsburgh and a licensed clinical psychologist. Dr. Molina conducts single- and multi-site study research on the course, causes, and treatments of ADHD and substance use/disorder amongst children and adults with increased risk and typical-healthy populations. She has concentrated on longitudinal studies of individuals with ADHD. Dr. Molina also studies stimulant misuse prevention via development of provider clinical practice strategies and longitudinal study of adolescents and young adults prescribed stimulants in primary care. Her program of research has been federally funded since 1995 including an NIH MERIT award. She has experience working successfully with community health and education providers and community member partnerships. She directs the Youth and Family Research Program at the University of Pittsburgh (yfrp.pitt.edu), sits on multiple journal editorial boards, and is on the board, served as program chair, and is President-Elect for the American Professional Society for ADHD and Related Disorders.

KOFI OBENG, diagnosed with attention-deficit/hyperactivity disorder (ADHD) in his late twenties, has been supporting people with ADHD on this journey for most of his adult life. To gain more support for his ADHD and to help others with ADHD, he joined the Attention Deficit Disorder Association (ADDA) in 2019. Shortly after joining, he volunteered to co-facilitate ADDA's African American/Black Diaspora + ADHD Peer Support Group. Volunteering for this leadership position led him to volunteer for several critical projects at ADDA, eventually leading to his hire as ADDA's Executive Director. In this role, he uses his leadership skills, his background in organizational transformation, and insights gained from lived experience to advance ADDA's mission of helping adults with ADHD discover and reach their potential.

MARK OLFSON, M.D., M.P.H., the Dollard Professor of Psychiatry, Medicine and Law and professor of epidemiology at Columbia University and Research Psychiatrist at New York State Psychiatric Institute, seeks to identify gaps between clinical science and practice in behavioral health care including a focus on improving the treatment and outcome of adults and young people with serious mental illnesses and substance use disorders. He has brought attention to problems in the quality of assessment and management of children and adults with behavioral health disorders including an emphasis on neglected and underserved populations. He has characterized unmet need for mental health services, the flow of patients into mental health care, and evolving national mental health service practice patterns. Olfson, who reports no conflicts of interest, has received numerous federal and private foundation grants, and has authored more than 600 academic papers.

Jennifer D. Oliva, J.D., MBA, is professor of law and Val Nolan Faculty Fellow at the Indiana University Maurer School of Law, a research scholar at Georgetown Law's O'Neill Institute for National & Global Health Law, and a senior scholar with the UCSF/UC Law Consortium on Law, Science & Health Policy. Professor Oliva's research and teaching interests include health law and policy, privacy law, evidence, torts, and complex litigation. Her scholarship has been published by or is forthcoming in, among other publications, the *Virginia Law Review, California Law Review, Duke Law Journal, Northwestern University Law Review, UCLA Law Review,* and online companions to the *University of Chicago Law Review* and *New York University Law Review.* Professor Oliva has earned numerous awards for her scholarship, teaching, and service. She was selected as a 2019 Wiet Life Science Law Scholar by the Loyola University Beazley Institute for Health Law and Policy and a 2020 Health Law Scholar by the Saint Louis University Center for Health Law Studies and the American Society of Law, Medicine & Ethics. Professor Oliva was the recipient of the 2021 Health Law Community Service Award from the AALS Section on Law, Medicine, and Health Care and the Harry S. Truman Foundation honored her with the 2019 Truman Scholarship Foundation Ike Skelton Award for her commitment to public service.

Sunny Patel, M.D., M.P.H., is a child, adolescent, and adult psychiatrist, serving as a Senior Advisor for Children, Youth, and Families at the Substance Abuse and Mental Health Service Administration. Prior to SAMHSA, Patel was appointed a White House Fellow and served at the Department of Homeland Security. He completed specialty fellowship training in child and adolescent psychiatry at NYU and Bellevue Hospital. He trained in adult psychiatry at Cambridge Health Alliance and was a clinical fellow at Harvard Medical School. He received his M.D. from the Mayo Clinic, an M.P.H. from Harvard, and graduated with college and departmental honors from UCLA.

J. Russell Ramsay, Ph.D., ABPP, is a licensed psychologist specializing in the assessment and psychosocial treatment of adult attention-deficit/hyperactivity disorder (ADHD). Before retiring from the University of Pennsylvania in June 2023 to start his independent telepsychology practice, he was professor of clinical psychology and co-founder and clinical director of PENN's Adult ADHD Treatment & Research Program. He has served terms on the professional advisory boards of the major ADHD organizations and is on the editorial board of the Journal of Attention Disorders. He has lectured internationally and is widely published, including five books on adult ADHD (with the sixth due in 2024). His patient guidebook, *The Adult ADHD Tool Kit* has been published in Spanish, French, and Korean, and a German translation is in process; it is a recommended adult ADHD self-help book by the Association for Behavioral and Cognitive Therapies. Ramsay is a CHADD Hall of Fame inductee.

LARA ROBINSON, PH.D. M.P.H., is a Lead Health Scientist with the Child Development and Disabilities Branch in the National Center on Birth Defects and Developmental Disabilities (NCBDDD), Centers for Disease Control and Prevention (CDC). As lead of the Applied Research and Evaluation team, she oversees work on the epidemiology of, research around risk/protective factors, health promotion programs for, and policy/programmatic evaluation of attention-deficit/hyperactivity disorder (ADHD) and Tourette syndrome activities. She received her doctoral degree in Applied Developmental Psychology from the University of New Orleans and her Master of Public Health degree from Tulane University. She also completed postdoctoral integrative research training in integrative children's mental health at the Pennsylvania State University. Robinson is a member of National Academies of Sciences, Engineering, and Medicine Forum on Child Well-Being. Clinically, she has worked as an Early Intervention evaluator and as a mental health consultant for childcare centers.

JONATHAN RUBIN, M.D., MBA, is the CMO and Senior Vice President of R&D at Supernus Pharmaceuticals, Inc. Before joining Supernus in 2020, Dr. Rubin was CMO of Atentiv from 2018 to 2020, and a consultant to Chondrial Therapeutics from 2017 to 2018. From 2013 to 2017, Rubin was CMO of Alcobra, where he supervised the completion of two Phase III studies in attention-deficit/hyperactivity disorder (ADHD). From 2007 to 2013, Dr. Rubin was Medical Director of Clinical Development and Medical Affairs for Shire Pharmaceuticals, where he supported the company's ADHD portfolio. Prior to Shire, Rubin was in private practice as a Developmental-Behavioral and General Pediatrician for 16 years. He was a pediatric resident at Albert Einstein/Montefiore Hospital and a fellow in ambulatory pediatrics at Boston's Children Hospital. Rubin received his M.D. from the University of Connecticut School of Medicine, his MBA from the Columbia School of Business and his B.S. in molecular biophysics and biochemistry from Yale University.

JOSEPH SCHATZ, DNP, CRNP, PMHNP-BC, CARN-AP, is a psychiatric/mental health nurse practitioner who has been living with attention-deficit/hyperactivity disorder (ADHD) since (at least) kindergarten (which is when Mrs. M. suggested to his parents that he might benefit from repeating the grade to work on his social skills). He is the Director of Penn Nursing's PMHNP track and treats patients across the lifespan for conditions including ADHD. In his practice, he sees the biggest barriers to effective treatment as failure to recognize/address co-occurring trauma, failure to treat ADHD in individuals with a history of substance use disorder, and failure to diagnose ADHD in adults due to clinician discomfort. Oh, and prior authorizations. Especially prior authorizations.

LaTasha Seliby Perkins, M.D., is a board-certified family physician practicing in Washington, D.C., and served as the new physician director to the American Academy of Family Physicians Board of Directors. She remains active in leadership as the academy's media ambassador, promoting the voice of the family physician. She is assistant professor at the Georgetown University School of Medicine Department of Family Medicine, where she is the course director of Community-Based Learning and chair of the DC AHEC Primary Care Mentorship Program. Seliby Perkins works clinically at MedStar Primary Care at Fort Lincoln Clinic Georgetown Family Residency Program, where she provides comprehensive care to patients of all ages. She spent eight years providing care to students at Georgetown University's Student Health Center.

Margaret Sibley, Ph.D., is a professor of psychiatry and behavioral sciences at the University of Washington School of Medicine and a clinical psychologist at Seattle Children's Hospital. She has authored more than 120 scholarly publications on attention-deficit/hyperactivity disorder (ADHD) across the lifespan with a current research portfolio funded by the National Institute of Mental Health and the Institute of Education Sciences. She is an investigator on the Multimodal Treatment of ADHD (MTA) Study, secretary of the American Professional Society for ADHD and Related Disorders (APSARD), a professional advisory board member for Children and Adults with Attention Deficit Hyperactivity Disorder (CHADD), the Diagnosis and Screening Subcommittee Chair for the APSARD Guidelines for Adult ADHD, and associate editor of the *Journal of Attention Disorders*.

Marta Sokolowska, Ph.D., is the Deputy Center Director for Substance Use and Behavioral Health in FDA's Center for Drug Evaluation and Research (CDER). She serves as the center's executive-level leader responsible for advancing FDA's public health response to the non-medical use of substances with abuse potential. With expertise in science-based assessment and management of drug abuse risks, Sokolowska advises senior FDA officials on shaping scientific and policy interventions and executing strategies pertaining to the use of controlled substances and behavioral health programs. She joined CDER in 2018 as Associate Director for Controlled Substances in the Office of the Center Director. Prior to joining FDA, Sokolowska held senior clinical and medical leadership roles in the pharmaceutical industry. She earned her doctoral degree in psychology from McMaster University in Canada.

MARY SOLANTO, PH.D., is professor of pediatrics and psychiatry at the Zucker School of Medicine at Hofstra-Northwell (Long Island, New York). Prior to joining Hofstra, she was director of the attention-deficit/hyperactivity disorder (ADHD) Center at the Mount Sinai School of Medicine and associate professor of psychiatry at NYU. In 2017–2018, Solanto was a Fulbright U.S. Scholar in the Netherlands where she conducted research on treatment of ADHD in college students, Dr. Solanto developed a novel cognitive-behavioral intervention for adults with ADHD, which was the focus of a NIMH-sponsored efficacy study (*American Journal of Psychiatry*, 2010). With her Co-PI, Dr. Anthony Rostain, Dr. Solanto most recently received NIMH funding to revise, refine, and test the CBT intervention for the needs of college students with ADHD.

BRANDI WALKER, PH.D., is the CEO of Marie Pauline Consulting, LLC, her private practice dedicated to providing educational, clinical, and psychological guidance and expertise to organizations seeking to improve their social climate and enhance their diversity and equity awareness. She is a licensed clinical psychologist, board-certified executive leadership coach, diversity and equity trainer, and organizational consultant on mental wellness and strategic planning. Walker is a Howard University and University of Maryland, alumna and a recently retired Army officer and faculty member at Womack Army Medical Center at Fort Liberty, North Carolina. Walker spent the last (7) years working with various hospitals/clinics, and schools conducting research on children with attention-deficit/hyperactivity disorder (ADHD), their family, and various sleep variables and environmental factors. She collaboratively initiated Prince George's County (Maryland) CHADD Chapter and the Southern Regional Support Center. Additionally, she currently conducts research with the Henry Jackson Foundation.

SARA WEISENBACH, PH.D. ABPP, is the Chief of Neuropsychology at McLean Hospital, a member of the faculty at Harvard Medical School, a board-certified clinical neuropsychologist, and a clinical translational researcher. Her career has been based on improving the quality of life for individuals with cognitive and psychiatric concerns through clinical care and innovation, cutting-edge research, education and mentorship, and service to the fields of Neuropsychology and Geriatric Psychiatry. She has been continuously funded since 2008 (NIH, VA) for her work on depression and cognition during middle-age and late life. Weisenbach earned her Ph.D. in Counseling Psychology from Colorado State University in 2005. She then went on to complete two post-doctoral fellowships; one in Clinical and Research Neuropsychology at University of Michigan and a second Special Fellowship in Geriatrics at the VA Ann Arbor Healthcare System. Weisenbach is a nationally recognized expert in cognitive and emotional health in older adults. She has developed stepped-care models for clinical evaluation of dementia and adult attention-deficit/hyperactivity disorder (ADHD). She is President for the Society for Clinical Neuropsychology of the American Psychological Association and Co-Chair of the Geriatric Mood Disorders Task Group of the National Network of Depression Centers. She regularly serves as a reviewer for peer-reviewed journals and NIH and VA study sections.

ROBIN WEISS, M.D., has followed a long and winding path throughout her medical career. Following a residency in pediatrics at the Residency Program in Social Medicine in the Bronx in 1981, she and her husband ran a pediatric ward on the island of St. Vincent, West Indies. Returning to the United States, she completed a Robert Wood Johnson Fellowship at The Johns Hopkins School of Medicine and was lured by the former dean of her medical school, Fred Robbins, to work at the Institute of Medicine. During the eventful years between 1985 and 1991, she became Director of HIV/AIDS activities at the IOM. Later, Weiss did a second residency in psychiatry at Sheppard Pratt Hospital in Baltimore, and in 1995 established a private practice and became active in state and local health policy. She has published articles on psychiatry, science, and health policy in the *New York Times* and other publications.

STAFF BIOSKETCHES

CAROLYN K. SHORE, PH.D., is a senior program officer with the Board on Health Sciences Policy of the National Academies of Sciences, Engineering, and Medicine (the National Academies). She is staff director of the Forum on Drug Discovery, Development, and Translation. Before joining the National Academies, Dr. Shore was an officer on Pew's antibiotic resistance project, leading work on research and policies to spur the discovery and development of urgently needed antibacterial therapies. She previously served as a foreign affairs officer at the U.S. Department of State, where she led an initiative on open data and innovation-based solutions to global challenges. She also served as the State Department's representative to intergovernmental organizations focusing on food safety, plant and animal health, biosecurity, and agricultural trade policy. Previously, Dr. Shore was an American Society for Microbiology congressional fellow, working on science-based policy related to antibiotic stewardship and other public health issues. She holds a doctoral degree in Microbiology and Molecular Genetics from Harvard University. As a graduate student, she studied anti-malarial drug resistance in Senegal and worked jointly between the Medicines for Malaria Venture, Genzyme Corporation, and the Broad Institute of Harvard and MIT to discover new anti-malarial compounds. Dr. Shore was awarded a Fulbright Fellowship for work at the University of Queensland in Brisbane, Australia, and a National Institutes of Health Training Grant for postdoctoral work at the University of Iowa.

SHEENA POSEY NORRIS, M.S., PMP, is a senior program officer on the Board on Health Sciences Policy at the National Academies of Sciences, Engineering, and Medicine's Health and Medicine Division. In this capacity, she serves as the Director of the Forum on Neuroscience and Nervous System Disorders, which brings together leaders from government, academia, industry, and non-profit organizations to discuss key challenges and emerging issues in neuroscience research, development of therapies for nervous system disorders, and related ethical and societal issues. She has led the planning of numerous workshops and activities in the areas of basic, translational, and clinical neuroscience; bioethics; training and workforce development; global mental health; and biodetection. In addition, she served as a staff officer on the Care Interventions for Individuals with Dementia and Their Caregivers and Preventing Dementia and Cognitive Impairment consensus studies. Prior to joining the National Academies, Posey Norris worked in the Graduate School of Nursing at the Uniformed Services University of the Health Sciences in Bethesda, Maryland. Working alongside advanced practice nurse researchers, she conducted research focusing on health promoting behaviors of military spouses. Posey Norris received her M.S. from Saint Joseph's University in Philadelphia, Pennsylvania, in experimental psychology with an emphasis in neuropsychology. Her thesis-driven research during her graduate studies focused on the neurocognitive and balance effects of multiple concussions in young adults. Posey Norris graduated magna cum laude from Lynchburg College in Virginia with a Bachelor of Science degree in psychology and Spanish (high honors).

KELSEY R. BABIK, M.P.H., CIH, is an associate program officer in the Health Medicine Division at the National Academies of Sciences, Engineering, and Medicine. In addition to this workshop, she works on projects initiated by the Committee on Personal Protective Equipment for Workplace Safety and Health. This is a standing committee at the National Academies of Sciences, Engineering, and Medicine sponsored by the National Personal Protective Technology Laboratory of the National Institute for Occupational Safety and Health, to provide a forum for discussion of scientific and technical issues relevant to the development, certification, deployment, and use of personal protective equipment, standards, and related systems to ensure workplace safety and health. Previously, at the Risk Sciences and Public Policy Institute of the Johns Hopkins Bloomberg School of Public Health, she worked on occupational health risk assessments for first responders. She is a certified industrial hygienist, has a B.S. in molecular biology from the University of Pittsburgh, an M.P.H. from the University of Maryland, and is currently pursuing a doctorate of public health (Dr.P.H.) at the University of Illinois Chicago.

NOAH ONTJES, M.A., is an associate program officer with the Board on Health Sciences Policy of the National Academies of Sciences, Engineering, and Medicine. He currently staffs the Forum on Drug Discovery, Development, and Translation, co-leading projects on engaging community practices in clinical trials and preparing the future workforce in drug R&D. He attended Wake Forest University where he graduated with a Bachelor of Science in biology and a triple minor in bioethics, chemistry, and psychology. His interest in the multiple factors that influence one's health paired with his love of different perspectives led him to pursue a Master of Arts in bioethics at Wake Forest University. During graduate school, he successfully defended his thesis on the reasonable person standard of disclosure in genetic research as well as collaborated on a published paper concerning the ethical considerations of electroconvulsive therapy on incapacitated patients.

MELVIN JOPPY, B.S., is a senior program assistant on the Board on Health Sciences Policy of the National Academies of Sciences, Engineering, and Medicine. He previously served as a Program Assistant at the Department of Energy (DOE) in the Office of Basic Energy Sciences. Prior to DOE, he served as the Committee Manager for the Presidential Advisory Council on HIV/AIDS (PACHA) within the U.S. Department of Health and Human Services. Joppy received his B.S. in communications from Bowie State University.